Strengthening the Palestinian Health System

Michael Schoenbaum · Adel K. Afifi · Richard J. Deckelbaum

Supported by a gift from David and Carol Richards

The research described in this report was funded by a gift from David and Carol Richards. This research in the public interest was also supported by RAND, using discretionary funds made possible by RAND's donors and the fees earned on client-funded research. This research was conducted under the direction of RAND Health's Center for Domestic and International Health Security in consultation with the RAND Center for Middle East Public Policy (CMEPP). RAND Health and CMEPP are units of the RAND Corporation.

Library of Congress Cataloging-in-Publication Data

Schoenbaum, Michael.
    Strengthening the Palestinian health system / Michael Schoenbaum, Adel K. Afifi, Richard J. Deckelbaum.
        p. cm.
    "MG-311."
    Includes bibliographical references.
    ISBN 0-8330-3730-7 (pbk. : alk. paper)
    1. Health planning—Palestine. 2. Medical policy—Palestine. 3. Medical care—Palestine.
    [DNLM: 1. Delivery of Health Care—organization & administration—Middle East. 2. Arabs—ethnology—Middle East. 3. Program Development—Middle East. W 84 JA2 S365s 2004] I. Afifi, Adel K. II. Deckelbaum, Richard J. III. Rand Corporation. IV. Title.

RA395.P19S35 2005
362.1'095695'3—dc22

2004028311

The RAND Corporation is a nonprofit research organization providing objective analysis and effective solutions that address the challenges facing the public and private sectors around the world. RAND's publications do not necessarily reflect the opinions of its research clients and sponsors.

RAND® is a registered trademark.

Cover design by Stephen Bloodsworth
Cover photo: "The Olive Tree: Hi Mama, I'm Home!"
Photographer: Steve Sabella at www.sabellaphoto.com

Published 2005 by the RAND Corporation
1776 Main Street, P.O. Box 2138, Santa Monica, CA 90407-2138
1200 South Hayes Street, Arlington, VA 22202-5050
201 North Craig Street, Suite 202, Pittsburgh, PA 15213-1516
RAND URL: http://www.rand.org/
To order RAND documents or to obtain additional information, contact Distribution Services: Telephone: (310) 451-7002;
Fax: (310) 451-6915; Email: order@rand.org

Preface

In June 2002, President Bush expressed U.S. support for creating an independent Palestinian state. At that time, he called for the establishment of an independent Palestinian state within three years; to this end, the United States joined the European Union, Russia, and the United Nations to pursue the "Roadmap" initiative in 2003.[1] Also in 2003, the Israeli government formally endorsed the eventual creation of an independent Palestinian state.

When President Bush made his initial declaration, the Roadmap was designed to meet a three-year timetable. At the time of this writing, however, the prospect of an independent Palestine by 2005 seems unlikely.[2] Nevertheless, a critical mass of Palestinians and Israelis—as well as the United States, Russia, the European Union, and the United Nations—remain committed to the establishment of a Palestinian state.

This study examines strategies for strengthening the health system of a potential independent Palestinian state. Successful development of the Palestinian health system is worthwhile in its own right, and it may be a relatively cost-effective way to help demonstrate the tangible benefits of independence and peaceful relations with neighboring countries. Moreover, implementation of many of the strategies described here can begin prior to independence. Research for this study was mainly conducted between December 2002 and July 2003. This study represents one component of a broader RAND Corporation analysis of options for structuring the institutions of a potential Palestinian state; all of the components are included in *Building a Successful Palestinian State*.[3]

---

[1] The full title of the Roadmap is "A Performance-Based Roadmap to a Permanent Two-State Solution to the Israeli-Palestinian Conflict" and can be found at: http://www.state.gov/r/pa/prs/ps/2003/20062pf.htm (dated April 30, 2003; available as of October 2004).

[2] Indeed, as this book went to press, President Bush called for establishing a Palestinian state before he leaves office in 2009.

[3] The RAND Palestinian State Study Team, *Building a Successful Palestinian State,* Santa Monica, Calif.: RAND Corporation, MG-146-DCR, 2005.

This study should be of interest to Palestinians and Israelis; to the international community, including the "Quartet"—the United States, the European Union, the United Nations, and Russia—that developed the "Roadmap" initiative; and to organizations and individuals committed to strengthening health and health care for Palestinians.

Funding for the project was provided by a generous gift from David and Carol Richards. This research in the public interest was also supported by RAND, using discretionary funds made possible by the generosity of RAND's donors and the fees earned on client-funded research. This research was conducted under the direction of RAND Health's Center for Domestic and International Health Security in consultation with the RAND Center for Middle East Public Policy (CMEPP). RAND Health and CMEPP are units of the RAND Corporation.

Contents

Figures and Tables

Figures

Tables

Summary

This book examines potential strategies for strengthening the Palestinian health system. We focus particularly on major institutions that would be essential for the success of the health system over the first decade of a future independent Palestinian state. In addition, we recommend several programs for preventive and curative care that are urgently needed and that could be implemented in the short term, with the goal of rapidly improving the health status and health care services of Palestinians.

The health system of a future Palestinian state starts with many strengths. These include a relatively healthy population; a high societal value placed on health; many highly qualified, experienced, and motivated health professionals, including clinicians, planners, administrators, technicians, researchers, and public health workers; national plans for health system development; and a strong base of governmental and nongovernmental institutions.

At the same time, there are important areas of concern. These include poor system-wide coordination and implementation of policies and programs, across geographic areas and between the governmental and nongovernmental sectors of the health system; many underqualified health care providers; weak systems for licensing and continuing education; and considerable deficits in the operating budgets of the Palestinian Ministry of Health and the government health insurance system (the principal source of health insurance). There are also important and persistent health problems, including gastroenteric and parasitic diseases, hepatitis A, respiratory infections, and meningitis; high—and rising—rates of malnutrition; and rising rates of chronic disease. Also, access to health care has declined, along with social and economic conditions, since the start of the second intifada in 2000.

This book describes a number of ways to strengthen the Palestinian health system, to help achieve specific health targets and financial sustainability. Our principal recommendations are as follows:

- Integrate health system planning and policy development more closely, with meaningful input from all relevant governmental and nongovernmental stakeholders.

- Develop viable and sustainable health insurance and health care financing systems.
- Update, standardize, and enforce licensing standards for all types of health care professionals.
- Update, standardize, and enforce standards for licensing and accrediting health care facilities and services.
- Improve training of health professionals, including academic and vocational training programs that are internationally accredited, and implement comprehensive and ongoing programs for continuing medical education.
- Implement a national strategy on health care quality improvement. Systematically evaluate quality improvement projects; disseminate those that succeed.
- Develop and enforce national standards for the licensing, supply, and distribution of pharmaceuticals and medical devices.
- Improve health information systems for tracking data such as health and nutritional status, use and costs of inpatient and outpatient care, health care quality, health system staffing, pharmaceutical inventories, health insurance enrollment, and medical records.
- Improve research and evaluation capacity, including public health, clinical, and biomedical research.
- Improve public and primary health care programs, including an updated immunization program, comprehensive micronutrient fortification and supplementation, prevention and treatment of chronic and noninfectious disease, and treatment of developmental and psychosocial conditions.

While all of these recommendations are important, we suggest that immediate priority be given to the first (improving system-wide coordination and implementation) and the last (improving public and primary health care programs).

In practice, the appropriate strategies for addressing these issues will depend on many factors that are currently unknown, including the borders of a future Palestinian state, its security arrangements and relations with its neighbors, its governance structure, and economic conditions. We therefore discuss policy alternatives applicable to several possible scenarios.

We believe that local stakeholders can and should determine both the overall development process and the details of the health system, particularly given the expertise that already exists in Palestine and among Palestinians living abroad. At the same time, we recognize that successful health system development in Palestine will require considerable outside resources, including technical and financial assistance. We estimate that the Palestinian health system could constructively absorb between $125 million and $160 million per year in external international support over the first decade of an independent state. For comparison, external support for the Palestinian health system averaged around $40 million per year over the period 1994–2000.

Successful development of the Palestinian health system is worthwhile in its own right, and it may be a relatively cost-effective way to help demonstrate the tangible benefits of independence and peaceful relations with neighboring countries. Moreover, health system development is an area where Israel, other neighboring countries, and the larger international community could play a constructive role, especially in areas such as health system planning, licensing and accreditation, development of information systems, and research.

Acknowledgments

We are grateful to Timea Spitka, who served as our project coordinator in Jerusalem; Nicole Lurie and C. Ross Anthony, who served as senior advisors; Meredith L. Magner, who provided research assistance; and Mechelle Wilkins, who provided administrative support. We would not have been able to conduct this work without them. We are also grateful for input and helpful comments on this book from Osman Galal, Shimon Glick, Laurie Brand, Ami Wennar, and several Palestinian and Israeli colleagues (who are not named here for reasons of confidentiality).

CHAPTER ONE

Introduction

Envisioning a successful Palestinian health system is a broad and challenging mandate. Therefore, we started by defining a scope of work that would be both feasible and useful—one that could provide constructive new information to Palestinian stakeholders and other interested parties. We decided to focus primarily on key "macro-level" programs and institutions that we consider to be prerequisites for developing, operating, and sustaining a successful national health system in Palestine. These include policies and programs covering health system planning and coordination across regions and stakeholders; licensing and accreditation of health professionals, facilities, and educational programs; human resource development; health insurance and health care financing programs; pharmaceutical policy; research and evaluation programs; health information systems; disease prevention and health promotion; and public health. We believe that responsibility for the "micro-level" details of health system organization, infrastructure, and operation properly rests with the local stakeholders, including the Palestinian Ministry of Health, the United Nations Relief and Works Agency for Palestinian Refugees in the Near East, relevant private and nongovernmental organizations, and, ultimately, Palestinian consumers who use health care services.

To date, Palestinian stakeholders have produced two detailed national health plans, the first in 1994, published by the Palestinian Council of Health (1994), the second in 1999, published by the Ministry of Health (PA MOH, 1999). These two plans had similar structures, approaches, and goals. (Indeed, many of the goals of the first were repeated in the second because they had not been fully achieved.) The 1999 plan covered the period 1999–2003 and is currently being updated. These national health plans were complemented by the *National Plan for Human Resource Development and Education in Health,* completed in 2001 by the Ministry of Health, the Ministry of Higher Education (now the Ministry of Education and Higher Education), and the Welfare Association (Welfare Association, PA, and Ministry of Higher Education, 2001a–f).[1]

---

[1] One of the authors of this book, Adel Afifi, was overall project coordinator for the development of the *National Plan for Human Resource Development and Education in Health.*

In part, these plans address system-wide development issues for Palestine, and we drew on this information extensively for our analyses. The national health plans also provide micro-level targets in many areas; e.g., the number, type, and geographic distribution of primary care clinics and different types of health care providers. Sample objectives from the 1999 national strategic health plan and the 2001 national plan for human resource development are included in Appendix A of this book.

Although we regard the micro-level targets as generally appropriate, it is beyond the scope of this project to affirm their validity. Similarly, we did not perform detailed assessments of prevailing standards of care or quality of care, conduct salary surveys for health care workers in the government sector, assess the suitability of various pilot systems or programs as national models, or conduct similar analyses of particular health system details.

The health system of a future Palestinian state starts with many strengths. These include a relatively healthy population, compared with other countries in the region with similar levels of economic development; many highly qualified, experienced, and motivated health professionals, including clinicians, planners, administrators, technicians, researchers, and public health workers; and a strong base of local institutions. At the same time, there are a number of opportunities to strengthen the Palestinian health system to achieve specific health targets and financial sustainability over time.

Successful development of the Palestinian health system is worthwhile in its own right. It may also be a relatively cost-effective way to help demonstrate tangible benefits of peace. Historically, the health sector has benefited from considerable and ongoing cooperation between Palestinian and Israeli institutions and individuals, in areas such as policy formation and human resource development. Despite the current tensions in the region, we found high levels of support on both sides for continuing and strengthening such cooperation as circumstances permit. If done with appropriate sensitivity to local needs and preferences, and with respect for the extensive infrastructure of Palestinian institutions that is already in place, health system development could also be an area where outside parties—including the United States—could play a constructive role. On the other hand, the social and political costs of neglecting health system development may be significant, particularly given Palestinians' high expectations regarding health and health care.[2]

In the following chapters of this book, we discuss the goals of a successful Palestinian health system. We describe our methods for conducting the health system analysis and provide brief background information on health and health care in the West Bank and Gaza. The remainder of the book presents specific recommendations for strengthening (and, in some cases, establishing) institutions and programs to promote the current and future success of the Palestinian health system. We conclude with a

---

[2] One factor affecting these expectations is Palestinians' proximity to and experience with the Israeli health system.

discussion of costs—the investment that will most likely be required to sustain a successful Palestinian health care system in the first decade of independence.

For ease of exposition, we refer to the West Bank and Gaza as "Palestine." When we discuss Jerusalem, we refer to it explicitly. We refer to the Ministry of Health of the Palestinian Authority as "the Ministry of Health," abbreviated as MOH. We use "the Palestinian government" to refer generically to the current and future governments of Palestine; when we mean the Palestinian Authority, abbreviated as PA, we refer to it explicitly. We abbreviate the United Nations Relief and Works Agency for Palestinian Refugees in the Near East as UNRWA.

In our discussion, we refer frequently to primary, secondary, and tertiary health care. Primary care refers to basic health care that is traditionally provided by physicians trained in family practice, internal medicine, or pediatrics, or by nonphysician providers such as nurses. Secondary care refers to care provided by specialty providers (e.g., urologists and cardiologists) who generally do not have first contact with patients; these providers usually see patients after referral from a primary or community health professional. Tertiary care refers to care provided by highly specialized providers (e.g., neurologists, cardiac surgeons, and intensive care units) in facilities equipped for special investigation and treatment.

All monetary figures are in nominal U.S. dollars (i.e., dollars that are not adjusted for inflation), unless otherwise noted.

CHAPTER TWO

What Is a Successful Health System?

A "successful" Palestinian health system should, at a minimum,

- maintain an effective and well-regulated public health system
- provide reasonable access to high-quality preventive and curative services for all Palestinians
- maintain high-quality programs for training health professionals
- achieve health outcomes at the population level that meet or exceed international guidelines, such as those recommended by the World Health Organization (WHO)
- be effective, efficient, and financially viable
- contribute to peace and encompass the possibility of cooperation with neighboring countries on issues of common interest.

There are many ways to achieve these broad goals, ranging from incremental reform to radical redesign. The two national health plans (1994 and 1999) and the *National Plan for Human Resource Development and Education in Health* (2001) articulate a vision of how the health system should develop over time, based mainly on incremental rather than radical change. This vision emphasizes public and primary health care as the "cornerstone" of service delivery, with expanded emphasis on health promotion and disease prevention capabilities. The public and primary care systems would be complemented by high-quality secondary and tertiary care systems, but these systems would be developed very carefully, and in a coordinated fashion, to ensure both clinical efficacy and economic efficiency.

In our view, this general vision conforms to the economic realities facing Palestine and to the available evidence from other settings regarding cost-effective health system development. We therefore adopted a similar focus on incremental reforms. In particular, we assume that the government will continue to be responsible for public health, a major provider of health care services; and a major, if not the primary, sponsor of health insurance over at least the first decade of an independent state.[1]

---

[1] In interviews with Palestinian stakeholders conducted as part of this analysis, some people expressed support for a transfer of the government's current health care delivery systems and health insurance programs to nongovernmental organizations (NGOs) or the private sector, which would leave the MOH responsible for planning, regulation, public health, provision for the indigent, and other functions for which the private sector is not well suited. Our recommendations do not foreclose such options. However, we think that these decisions must be made locally.

CHAPTER THREE

Alternative Scenarios for an Independent State

Our mandate is to describe strategies for strengthening the Palestinian health system to support the success of a future independent Palestinian state. However, the essential characteristics of the future state are currently unknown. In practice, characteristics such as the state's borders, security arrangements, and relations with its neighbors will significantly affect health system development. For this analysis, we therefore consider several possible scenarios for the characteristics of a future state, and we discuss how our policy recommendations might change for each scenario.

Population Mobility

Over the last several years, travel by Palestinians within the West Bank, between the West Bank and Gaza, and to East Jerusalem has frequently been restricted, particularly since the start of the second intifada in September 2000 and with the construction of Israel's separation barrier. Lack of mobility—for people and supplies—has limited patient and provider access to health care facilities, limited the collection of epidemiological and other health-related data, and been associated with declines in nutritional status, among other effects. The geographic closures have been sufficiently long-lasting that all stakeholders in the health system have taken active steps to minimize the short-term consequences, for instance by building new local treatment facilities to help meet the acute needs of patients who would have traveled for care under less restrictive conditions.[1]

For purposes of the future health system, the relevant issue is the degree of population mobility that will be possible within a future Palestinian state. We consider two possible scenarios:

---

[1] There has also been some damage to relevant infrastructure, particularly in conjunction with Israeli military operations in the West Bank during and after March 2002.

- *Unrestricted Domestic Mobility.* This scenario assumes free movement within the West Bank and within Gaza in a future independent Palestinian state. In general, it also assumes that patients would be able to travel between the West Bank and Gaza. Because these areas are relatively distant from each other, primary and secondary care would probably be handled within each area; travel to another area would become important if the patient is referred to a tertiary care center. Similarly, although the status of East Jerusalem is uncertain, we assume that Palestinians will have relatively open access to health care facilities in East Jerusalem.
- *Restricted Domestic Mobility.* This scenario assumes that movement within and between the territories of a future Palestinian state will be restricted (or, in the extreme case, prevented). Various factors could limit mobility, including the degree of territorial contiguity and Palestinian and Israeli security policies. Except as noted, health system development strategies do not depend on the specific cause of mobility restrictions, only on their scope and duration.

In practice, we regard free movement of patients, health professionals, and supplies within Palestine as prerequisites for successful health system development and operation. Restricted mobility would perpetuate and magnify the problems of staffing, supply, and patient access that have prevailed in the Palestinian health system during the second intifada. Moreover, strategies to mitigate these problems would be clinically and economically inefficient, relative to development under free mobility, particularly because the problems inhibit the development and operation of regional referral centers.

As a result, we consider unrestricted domestic mobility to be the default scenario for our analyses. However, at the end of each substantive subsection, we discuss how our recommendations would change under conditions of restricted mobility.

International Access[2]

The extent to which travel is restricted between an independent Palestinian state and other countries, particularly Israel and Jordan, may also significantly affect the future health system. We consider two possible scenarios:

- *Unrestricted Access.* This scenario assumes that Palestinians face no categorical restrictions on travel to Israel, Jordan, or elsewhere for purposes of receiving health care or for professional training.

---

[2] Here, "access" refers to the right to travel to and stay in foreign countries, rather than insurance coverage or other factors that affect whether foreign institutions will accept Palestinian patients. As with domestic mobility, international access is likely to be contingent on successful security arrangements.

- *Restricted Access.* This scenario assumes that access for Palestinians to Israel, Jordan, and elsewhere for purposes of receiving health care or professional training is significantly restricted.

Unrestricted access is clearly preferable for health system development, because it provides additional options for meeting clinical and educational needs. As a result, we consider unrestricted access to be the default scenario for our analyses. However, at the end of each substantive subsection, we discuss how our recommendations would change under conditions of restricted international access.

Other Cross-Cutting Issues

Other characteristics of a future independent state will also affect health system development in important ways. For instance, any successful health system development depends on effective governance. This extends to all branches of government—i.e., the executive, legislative, and judicial branches. Effective development will also require meaningful inclusion of nongovernmental stakeholders in health system planning, policymaking, and policy implementation.

Successful security arrangements between Israel and Palestine are crucial to the successful development of Palestinian institutions. Continued conflict between the two states would, among other consequences, reduce the willingness of international donors to commit staff, money, and other resources to support health system projects; reduce the supply of private capital available for health system development from both local and international sources; encourage emigration of skilled and educated health professionals; and constrain public and private budgets.

Any successful health system development is also contingent on the financial resources available. As we discuss in detail in Chapter Eight, a Palestinian health system that can truly be viewed as "successful" along the lines envisioned by our mandate will require considerable outside investment over at least the first decade of independence. The amount of outside resources and the period of time for which they are required depend on the performance of the Palestinian economy. Improved economic conditions will increase the level of both public and private resources available locally. Improved economic and social conditions are also associated with improved population health outcomes, independent of health care use.

For ease of exposition, we do not define specific scenarios for these additional characteristics. However, we considered them in all our analyses and discuss their effects on our recommendations, as appropriate.

CHAPTER FOUR

Methods

This book presents independent analyses conducted by the authors. Information about the Palestinian health system came from published and unpublished analyses by government organizations (e.g., the Palestinian and Israeli Ministries of Health), reports by international organizations (e.g., World Bank, various United Nations agencies, and the WHO), reports by Palestinian and international nongovernmental organizations (NGOs), papers in scientific journals, conference proceedings, working papers, and other formats. We did not collect new quantitative data.

We interviewed many Palestinian, Israeli, and international stakeholders who were experienced with and knowledgeable about, and in many cases have or had responsibility for, important aspects of the Palestinian health system. Interviews were primarily conducted in person during a trip to Palestine and Israel in May 2003. We asked all interview participants to allow themselves to be identified in this book. However, to help ensure that people felt free to express their views fully, interview participants were assured that no comments would be quoted directly or attributed to them in an identifiable way.

Study methods are described in further detail in Appendix B, which also includes an alphabetical list of interview participants. The letter of introduction we sent to local stakeholders is included in Appendix C.

As we began this project, we learned that the European Union was sponsoring a comprehensive health sector review on behalf of the Palestinian MOH. That review aims to analyze major areas of the health sector, to assess the constraints resulting from the intifada, and to suggest the elements for a refocused midterm health development strategy. Additional information about that review is included in Appendix D.

CHAPTER FIVE

Background

This chapter provides a brief overview of health and health care in Palestine. The information was drawn from a variety of sources, particularly Barnea and Husseini (2002); the annual reports of the Ministry of Health (e.g., PA MOH, 2002a); the first and second Palestinian national health plans (see PA MOH, 1999; Welfare Association, PA, and Ministry of Higher Education, 2001a–f); Giacaman, Abdul-Rahim, and Wick (2003); the scientific literature; and data compiled at the Health Inforum web site (http://www.healthinforum.net/).[1] These and other references are provided in the bibliography.

We note that systematic collection of health data has been difficult since the start of the second intifada; we therefore report the most current information available to us at the time of this writing.

Health Status

Life expectancy at birth in Palestine is about 70 years (as of 2000), higher than all neighboring countries except Israel. The infant mortality rate is approximately 23 per 1,000 live births, less than half the rate during the 1970s and comparable to or lower than rates in neighboring countries other than Israel (the Israeli rate is 6 per 1,000 live births). The maternal mortality rate was 19 per 100,000 births in 1998–1999, also down by more than half since 1980. The Palestinian maternal mortality rate is considerably better than those in Jordan, Iran, and Egypt, but some four times the Israeli and Kuwaiti rates (see Table 5.1).

Palestinian health indicators have improved significantly over time. Since the 1970s, standards of living and hygiene improved steadily, as did access to health care. For instance, the fraction of households with three or more people per room declined

---

[1] Health Inforum describes itself as the "information body linked directly with the Core Group of the Health Sector Working Group." It was formed in 2001 through the collaboration of the World Health Organization, the Italian Cooperation, USAID, Maram, UNSCO, and UNDP.

Table 5.1
Basic Health Indicators, Palestine and Elsewhere (1998–1999)

	Life Expectancy at Birth (years)	Infant Mortality Rate (per 1,000 live births)	Mortality Rate for Children Under Age 5 (per 1,000 live births)	Maternal Mortality Rate (per 100,000 live births)
Palestine	70	23	28	19
Israel	78	6	6	5
Jordan	68	30	36	41
Egypt	67	51	69	170
Kuwait	68	12	13	5
Qatar	72	15	18	10
Iran	69	29	33	37
Yemen	58	87	121	350
United States	77	7	8	8
France	78	5	5	10

SOURCES: United Nations Children's Fund, 2000; PA MOH, 2002a.

from 47 percent in 1975 to 28 percent in 1992 in the West Bank, and from 47 percent to 38 percent in Gaza. Similarly, by the mid-1990s, more than 90 percent of homes had electricity (up from around 25 percent in 1972–1975), and more than three-quarters of Palestinian households had access to clean, chlorinated drinking water (up from under one-quarter in 1972–1975). Access to primary health care services also improved significantly since 1970, as both the Israeli administration (before 1994) and the PA (from 1994 onward) expanded the number and geographic distribution of primary care and maternal and child health clinics.

Another factor contributing to lower infant mortality rates is the substantial expansion over time in the fraction of births occurring in a health facility or attended by a trained health professional: In 2001, 82 percent of Palestinian births occurred in a hospital, and 95 percent were attended by a health professional. The long-standing strength of the Palestinian immunization program also played an important role in improving child health. Immunization rates among children for the major vaccine-preventable diseases (e.g., polio, measles, mumps, rubella, diphtheria, tetanus, pertussis, and most recently hepatitis B) have exceeded 95 percent since the mid-1980s; as a result, incidence of these diseases has been low or zero since the 1980s. Also, from 1986 to 1998, infants and pregnant women attending government maternal and child health centers and village health rooms received vitamin and mineral supplements (iron and vitamins A and D for infants, and iron and folate for women). These supplements helped improve infant growth patterns and reduce malnutrition and susceptibility to infectious disease.

Some indicators, such as immunization coverage and the fraction of births occurring in medical facilities, have declined since the beginning of the second intifada, primarily because of travel restrictions for providers and patients. However, the magnitude of these changes is currently unknown.

Incidence of gastroenteric and parasitic diseases has also declined significantly since the 1980s, and outcomes have improved. However, these conditions remain important health problems, primarily because of hygienic conditions (which have deteriorated since the start of the second intifada). Other areas of concern include hepatitis A, which is endemic in Palestine; respiratory infections; and meningitis. To date, vaccines for hepatitis A, haemophilus influenza B, and varicella have not been added to the Palestinian immunization program.

Acute and chronic malnutrition are also relatively prevalent, as are anemia and other micronutrient deficiencies. Nutritional status has declined in the last few years, as measured by indicators such as anthropometric status of children, anemia levels, and reported nutrient intake. Factors that might contribute to declining nutritional status include declining economic conditions, particularly since the outbreak of the second intifada, and the cessation in 1998–1999 of routine vitamin and mineral supplementation for infants and pregnant women in the government health system.[2]

As the role of infectious disease has declined in Palestine, the relative importance of noncommunicable and chronic illness has risen. As in most countries, stroke, ischemic heart disease, hypertension, diabetes, and cancer together account for more than half of adult mortality, and incidence and prevalence rates for these conditions have been rising over time. Among infants and children, one-third of deaths are due to accidents (of all kinds), more than any other identifiable category of causes.

Health status in Palestine is described in detail elsewhere, particularly in annual reports published by the MOH. However, data regarding inequities in health status between rural and urban residence, between refugee and nonrefugee populations, and by geographic region are relatively limited. Our recommendations for improving data collection are discussed in Chapter Six.

Health System Organization

Before 1994

Prior to being occupied by Israel in 1967, Gaza was administered by Egypt, while the West Bank and East Jerusalem were administered by Jordan. Health institutions in each area operated independently from each other. Gaza followed Egyptian protocols for medical licensing and other relevant issues, while the West Bank followed Jordanian protocols.

---

[2] Declines in nutritional status have been documented in several recent studies, which differ primarily in their estimates of the magnitude of the decline. Another recent survey, conducted by the WHO, found that other health status indicators had not declined significantly during the second intifada but cautioned that such declines might be forthcoming if social and economic conditions continued to decline.

Between 1967 and 1994, these areas were both administered by the Israeli Defense Ministry. Gaza and the West Bank had separate chief medical officers and administrative structures, and they continued to follow different protocols in certain health policy areas, particularly those relating to medical licensing and supervision of health facilities. While many aspects of health policy were standardized for both the West Bank and Gaza, there were also some differences between the two areas, including differences in vaccination programs, maternal and child health programs, primary care services, and health insurance. As we discuss further below, the policy differences between Gaza and the West Bank remain relevant today.

Since 1948, UNRWA has been charged with providing basic health services to registered Palestinian refugees, including in the West Bank and Gaza. Refugees eligible for UNRWA services include those Palestinians (and their descendants) who were displaced from their homes because of the war between Israeli and Arab armies in 1948. Currently, approximately 75 percent of Gaza residents and 30 percent of West Bank residents—a total of some 1.5 million people in those areas—are designated as refugees. During most of the period of Israeli administration, UNRWA headquarters were in Vienna, Austria, and most planning for UNRWA health programs in Palestine was done there. UNRWA headquarters were subsequently moved to Amman, Jordan.

As described by some of its top Israeli managers, the objectives of the Israeli administration were to provide good health care, given the available resources; to minimize the risk of political unrest; and to provide a stable basis from which to negotiate a political solution.[3] The top managers of the government health system were Israeli physicians appointed by the Israeli Defense Ministry, with supervision from the Israeli Health Ministry. High-level planning was directed by the Israeli administration, generally via joint committees with senior Palestinian health officials. Most staff of the government health sector were Palestinian, including administrative and clinical personnel. Some independent review was provided by visiting experts from the WHO, the International Committee of the Red Cross, and other organizations.

Israel aimed at financial self-sufficiency of the government health sector. Approximately half of the total health budget came from Palestinian taxes (and health insurance premiums) during the 1970s, rising to 75–100 percent during the 1980s and early 1990s. Consistent with these financial goals, the government health system placed a heavy emphasis on public health and primary care, particularly immunization programs for vaccine-preventable illness, and maternal and child health programs. Between 1970 and 1993, the number of government maternal and child health clinics increased by 488 percent, while the number of general government clinics increased by 63 percent.

In contrast, relatively little capital investment was directed toward secondary and tertiary care. For instance, the number of government hospital beds in the West Bank

---

[3] These objectives are described by Yitzhak Sever and Yitzhak Peterburg in Barnea and Husseini (2002). Both served as chief medical officers with the Israeli Civil Administration, in the West Bank and Gaza, respectively.

and Gaza increased by just 13 percent between 1970 and 1993. Similarly, in 1992, approximately 10 percent ($5.9 million) of the government health budget for Palestine went to development; the rest went toward operating expenses.[4] Hospital development efforts were focused on strengthening personnel and capacity in key departments, particularly anesthesia and internal medicine; also, all regional hospitals developed fully operational renal dialysis units during this period, and several hospitals were developing tertiary care services such as cardiac and neurosurgery.

Transfer to the Palestinian Authority

Following the Oslo agreement in 1993, Israel and the Palestinians negotiated the transfer of responsibility for health services and health policy from Israeli administration to the newly formed PA. The PA assumed health sector responsibility for Gaza and Jericho in May 1994 and for the rest of the West Bank at the end of that year.

The Palestinian health system is commonly described as consisting of four "sectors": the government sector, led by the MOH; the private sector; the NGO sector; and the sector run by UNRWA. The MOH serves as the principal administrative and regulatory body for the Palestinian health system, although responsibility for some relevant areas is also held by other ministries, including the Ministry of Finance (e.g., for budgeting), the Ministry of Planning (e.g., for infrastructure development programs), and the Ministry of Education and Higher Education (for academic and vocational training programs). The MOH manages public health services and delivery of primary, secondary, and tertiary care in government facilities. The MOH organizational chart from the second Palestinian national health plan (published in 1999) is reproduced as Figure 5.1.

Health Care Infrastructure

Table 5.2 provides data on some key indicators of health system infrastructure and capacity in Palestine, along with some international comparisons. The role of the government sector in health care delivery—relative to that of the NGOs, private, and UNRWA sectors—is presented in Table 5.3.

---

[4] The Israeli administration published data on government health sector expenditures for the West Bank from 1990 ($26.7 million, $34 per capita) through 1993 ($37.2 million, $37 per capita). Relatively little public data were available for other periods, or for Gaza. Moreover, budget records were not among the information provided to the MOH by Israel when responsibility for the health system was transferred to the PA.

Figure 5.1
Ministry of Health Organizational Structure

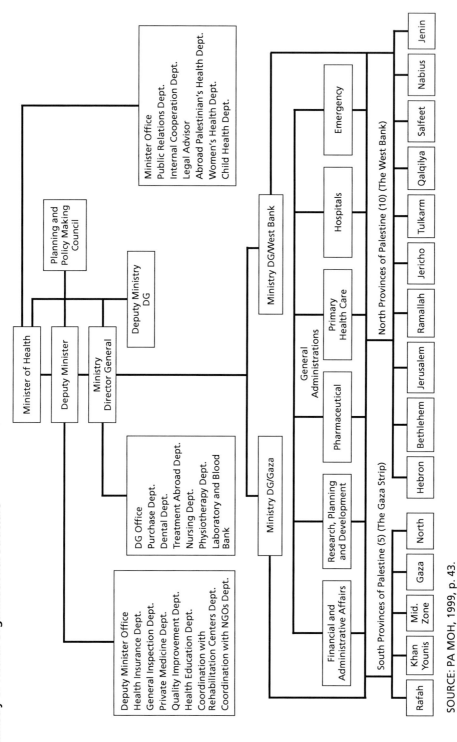

SOURCE: PA MOH, 1999, p. 43.
NOTE: Our understanding is that this organizational chart remains generally accurate, although some details may have changed since it was produced.
RAND MG311-5.1

Table 5.2
Health System Infrastructure, Palestine and Elsewhere (2000–2001, unless otherwise noted)

	Palestine	Israel	Jordan	Egypt	European Union	United States
GNP per capita	$1,771	$16,710	$1,650[c]	$1,080[c]	$22,363	$35,182
Health system spending per capita	$111[a]	$1,671	$139	$45[f]	$2,123	$4,887
Health system spending as a percentage of GNP	6%	10%	8%	4%[g]	10%	14%
Hospital beds per 100,000 population	137	614	160[d]	210[d]	622	360
Hospital occupancy rate	76.9%[b]	93%[b]	70%[g]	55%[e]	78%[b]	67%
Physicians per 100,000 population	84	377	165[d]	76	349	240
Nurses per 100,000 population	120	590	250[c]	N.A.	668	810
Dentists per 100,000 population	9	114	49[c]	6	64	60
Pharmacists per 100,000 population	10	62	N.A.	6	79	62

SOURCES: World Bank, 1998, 2003b; World Health Organization, 2001, 2004; The Hashemite Kingdom of Jordan, 2004; Gaumer et al., 1998; Medistat, 2003; Partnerships for Health Reform, 1997; PA MOH, 2002a; European Commission and Eurostat, 2001; Barnea and Husseini, 2002; Organisation for Economic Co-operation and Development, 1997, 2004; Centers for Disease Control and Prevention, 2003.

NOTE: N.A. = not available. As described elsewhere in this book, gross national product (GNP) per capita has since fallen substantially as a result of the second intifada.

[a] Data are from 1997.
[b] Occupancy rate is for MOH hospitals in Palestine and for acute care hospitals elsewhere.
[c] Data are from 1996.
[d] Data are from 1998.
[e] Data are for all hospitals in 1996.
[f] Data are for 2002.
[g] Data are for government hospitals in 1996; occupancy in private hospitals for that year was 49 percent.

Health System Funding and Expenditures

The annual operating budget for the MOH peaked at around $100 million in 1997 but has declined fairly continuously since then because of declining revenue from health insurance premiums and a general budget crisis. At least up to 2000 and the second intifada, government revenue for the health sector came from general taxation (60 percent), health insurance premiums (25–30 percent), and patient cost sharing (10–15 percent). In 1998, government health spending was $88 million, of which $39 million was spent on salaries, $25 million on drugs and medical supplies, $9 million on treatment abroad, and $14 million on other operating costs.[5]

---

[5] The component for salaries has been the largest, and fastest growing, part of MOH spending, with the number of MOH employees more than doubling between 1993 and 2001, from 4,020 to 8,285. This was driven in part by a doubling of the number of government outpatient clinics and increases in hospital capacity during this period.

Table 5.3
Distribution of Capacity Across the Sectors of the Palestinian Health System (2001)
(in percentage)

	Government	UNRWA	NGOs	Private
General hospital beds	53	1	37	10
Specialized hospital beds	75	N.A.	13	12
Maternity hospital beds	31	N.A.	33	37
Primary health clinics	61	8	30	N.A.
Health employees	56	7	30	7
Expenditures (1997)[a]	33	11	16[b]	40[c]

SOURCES: PA MOH, July 2002a; World Bank, 1998.
NOTE: N.A. = not available.
[a] Includes capital expenditures.
[b] Combines international donors and NGOs.
[c] Includes household expenditures and private capital investments.

Overall, Palestinian health system spending was estimated to be around $320 million in 1998, including infrastructure development.[6,7] In addition to the $88 million spent by the MOH, spending on health care in the private sector was approximately $90 million per year, while NGO spending on health care was estimated to be around $70 million.[8] UNRWA spending on health in Palestine was around $18 million in 1998.

The remainder of national health expenditures—some $54 million in 1998—came from other sources, particularly international donors.[9] Between mid-1994 and mid-2000, international donors disbursed approximately $227 million in health development assistance to Palestine, excluding humanitarian assistance. This averaged about $38 million per year, more than six times the governmental development budget during the last years of Israeli administration. Although detailed data on the distribution of international donations between infrastructure development and ongoing expenses

---

[6] We use 1998 as a reference point here because relatively detailed data were available to us for that year and because financing in subsequent years was significantly distorted by the second intifada. Additional information on health system spending is provided in Chapter Eight.

[7] Palestine spent approximately 6 percent of gross national product (GNP) on health in 1998. The fraction of GNP spent on health in Israel was somewhat higher (10 percent). More important, Israeli GNP per capita—and thus health spending per capita—was more than nine times higher than that in Palestine (World Bank, 1998; PA MOH, 2002a). Moreover, Palestinian national income and health system spending have fallen considerably since 2000; this is discussed further in Chapter Eight.

[8] Publicly available data on private-sector and NGO spending on health are limited, so these estimates may be somewhat inaccurate.

[9] All of these figures exclude East Jerusalem. Estimates for the amount contributed annually by Palestinians in East Jerusalem to Israeli national insurance—which includes health insurance—range from $30 million to $40 million.

are unavailable, donors have certainly preferred to direct donations toward the former, and they have been particularly reluctant to fund the operating expenses of the government sector. For example, of the $224 million in donor commitments made to health sector development to cover the period 1994–1997, only 5 percent ($12 million) was specifically designated for recurring costs; 24 percent of the total commitments was specifically designated for other purposes, mostly equipment and construction, while the designated purpose for the rest was mixed or unspecified.[10]

A schematic for the flow of funds in the health system is reproduced as Figure 5.2.

Patient Benefits and Costs

Government Health Benefits

Under PA administration, the entire Palestinian population, regardless of health insurance or refugee status, is entitled by statute and government policy to immunizations, prenatal and postnatal care, preventive and curative care for children until age three, basic preventive services, hospital care, and community mental health services, without patient cost sharing. The predominant source of health insurance in Palestine is currently the government insurance program, which covers primary, secondary, and tertiary curative care. Palestinians who officially reside in East Jerusalem (i.e., those with a Jerusalem identity card) participate in the compulsory Israeli health insurance programs and receive care under those systems. Participation in the government plan is mandatory for government (i.e., PA and municipal) workers and for Palestinians working in Israel. Other people may join the government program voluntarily as individuals, households, or groups organized around a firm or workplace.

The current government health insurance program is modeled closely on the system originally introduced by Israel. However, the MOH deliberately reduced insurance premiums after 1994 to promote enrollment. This strategy was generally effective: enrollment increased from 20 percent of households in 1993 to 55 percent in 1996. Enrollment subsequently declined because of a budget crisis in the government health sector and worsening economic conditions. However, premiums were recently waived for large segments of the population, particularly the households of people who lost jobs in Israel since the onset of the second intifada or who have been hurt in clashes with Israel, and enrollment has consequently increased.

Until the outbreak of the second intifada, health insurance premiums for government employees and participants via workplace groups were 5 percent of a worker's base monthly salary, with a monthly minimum of $8.50 and a maximum of $16.[11]

---

[10] We lack similar data on the distribution of actual disbursements, as opposed to donor commitments.

[11] Premiums and cost sharing are paid in Israeli shekels (NIS). Costs in U.S. dollars are based on a rate of $1 = 4.74 NIS, the rate at the end of March 2003.

Figure 5.2
Flow of Funds in Palestinian Health System

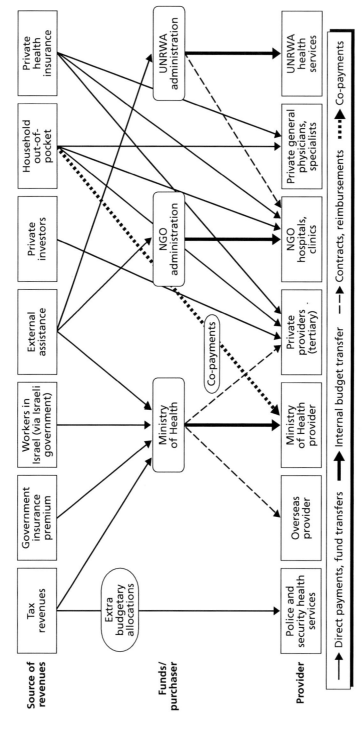

SOURCES: World Bank, 1998, p. 24. Also appears in Barnea and Husseini, 2002, p. 184.

NOTE: Several sets of arrows are missing from this figure. For instance, arrows should run from the MOH to NGOs and the private sector. As described below, government health benefits do not cover some care from such providers when patients are referred because a covered service is not available in the government system. Also, an arrow should run from UNRWA to the MOH. As also described below, UNRWA pays government insurance premiums for some UNRWA beneficiaries.

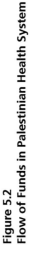

RAND MG311-5.2

Private participants were charged $10.50 per month for individual coverage and $16 for household coverage.[12] Palestinians working in Israel were charged $20 per month, a small part of which was deducted by Israel to pay for care provided there. Parents over age 60 could be covered for an additional $3 per month in premium payments. Health insurance premiums were waived for households that met "hardship" criteria, with the MOH assuming responsibility for them.[13]

When economic conditions declined significantly after the outbreak of the second intifada, enrollment in the government health system also fell. Correspondingly, the fraction of the MOH operating budget that came from health insurance premiums fell from 40 percent in 1999 to 24 percent in 2001. This revenue source was then substantially reduced when the PA decided to waive government health insurance premiums for large segments of the population, as a result of the emergency conditions associated with the second intifada.[14] As of this writing, insurance premiums remain waived.

Even for people whose premiums have been waived, some co-payments remain. Under the government health insurance program, patients are charged $0.21 per laboratory test and for imaging services. If a private provider refers patients to the government sector for care, patients are charged $4 per referral by the government insurance program, although apparently this charge is often not enforced. Pharmacy co-payments are described below. With the exception of these charges, there is no cost sharing for outpatient and inpatient care in the government sector under the government insurance plan, nor for care in the NGO or private sectors (or in foreign institutions) for patients who receive appropriate referrals from the government system. In theory, the government system pays for care in the NGO and private sectors only when an appropriate referral has been obtained. Referrals are supposed to be provided only when needed services are not available from government providers.

Under the pharmacy benefit of the government insurance program, patients are charged $0.63 per prescription for medications ($0.21 for children up to age three). Patients obtain prescription drugs from government clinics; in general, drugs obtained from private pharmacies are not covered by the government plan. The MOH developed a national essential drug list, which was released in 2002. In principle, all the drugs on the list—and only the drugs on the list—are available to patients in the gov-

---

[12] For comparison, Palestinian gross national income was around $1,800 per capita in 2000 and $1,070 per capita in 2002, based on data from the MOH.

[13] Hardship cases included indigent households and those that met certain other criteria, such as households headed by widows. In 1998, before the second intifada and the waiving of premiums for many people, approximately 20 percent of participants in the government health insurance system were hardship cases; 30 percent were required to participate as government employees; 20 percent were required to participate as workers in Israel; and 30 percent were enrolled on a voluntary basis, as individuals or via group contracts.

[14] Enrollment in the government insurance system increased again when premiums were waived, to some 80 percent of the population. However, the MOH budget has not been increased to fully reflect the associated liabilities for the government health system. We discuss health insurance in greater detail in Chapter Six.

ernment health sector. In practice, not all covered drugs are consistently available in all geographic areas, because of factors including insecure supply, poor distribution, and the MOH planning process. However, purchase of drugs from private pharmacies is not covered by the government health plan, even if the drugs were prescribed by but were unavailable in the government health system. We discuss pharmaceutical policy in greater detail in Chapter Six.

The MOH is the main provider of hospital beds, particularly in Gaza. The MOH is also the main provider of primary care, operating a large network of primary care clinics, maternal and child health centers, and village health rooms. Immunizations are provided by the MOH at its primary care sites and in UNRWA clinics, as well as via traveling immunization teams for areas that lack on-site services.

Health care providers in the government sector are salaried public employees. Providers in UNRWA and most NGOs are also salaried employees. Private practice has expanded since 1994 but is still fairly limited, especially in Gaza.

United Nations Relief and Works Agency

UNRWA's health services focus on disease prevention and control, primary care, family health, health education, physiotherapy, school health, psychosocial support services, and environmental health. There is no patient cost sharing for these services, which are provided mainly through a network of UNRWA outpatient clinics throughout the West Bank and Gaza, primarily in areas with significant concentrations of refugees. UNRWA also provides some secondary care; patients must pay 25 percent of the cost of care (10 percent in hardship cases) for these services, which are provided through one UNRWA hospital, in the West Bank, and in public and NGO hospitals with which UNRWA contracts for inpatient care. In general, UNRWA does not cover care for chronic and noncommunicable diseases. For some conditions, particularly cancer, UNRWA "sponsors" patients' care by covering the cost of enrolling the patient in the government health insurance program.

UNRWA's budget is determined by the United Nations General Assembly. However, in practice the budget allocation is not always fully funded by donor countries. For example, in 1998, donor countries provided $18 million (72 percent) out of an approved health budget of $25 million for Palestine.

Since this analysis is framed in terms of a future independent Palestinian state, it is worth commenting on the likely role of UNRWA in that context. Nearly all Palestinian stakeholders whom we interviewed thought that the role of UNRWA in Palestine would be eliminated with a final political settlement and the establishment of an independent state, and that the UNRWA system would probably be transferred to the MOH eventually.[15]

---

[15] Since UNRWA's services are financed by international donations, the MOH and donor countries would need to work together to ensure that such a transfer does not cause a financial shock to the Palestinian health system.

Use of UNRWA services does not affect eligibility for government health insurance and services.

NGOs and the Private Sector

Nongovernmental organizations have played a very important role in all levels of the Palestinian health system, during both the Israeli and Palestinian administrations. Although some international NGOs operate in Palestine, the role of indigenous NGOs is at least as great. NGOs include organizations with social, political, and religious motivations. Historically and today, NGOs in Palestine have provided services including outpatient and inpatient care, psychosocial support, rehabilitation, health education, and emergency care. They have also been active in health promotion and health education, consumer activism, health planning, infrastructure development, human resource development, and other aspects of the health system.

NGO development was particularly significant during the first intifada and the period immediately preceding the Oslo agreement (1987–1993), when NGOs were one feasible outlet for developing national institutions. Following the transfer of the health system to the MOH, international donors shifted substantial resources from the NGO sector to the government sector, a trend that was somewhat reversed following the start of the second intifada.

Private investment in the health sector was relatively limited before 1994 but grew considerably between 1994 and 2000. The private health sector now includes clinics and hospitals; pharmacies; laboratories; radiology, physiotherapy, and rehabilitation centers; and medical equipment manufacturing facilities. In addition, there is a growing domestic pharmaceutical industry, which produces approximately 700 different products and supplies a substantial amount—estimated to be around one-half—of the Palestinian demand for prescription drugs. There have been some attempts to establish private health insurance programs, but private coverage has never exceeded 2–3 percent of the population. Private insurance plans have essentially been eliminated by the economic hardships accompanying the second intifada. However, private expenditures on health remain considerable (see Table 5.3).[16]

---

[16] The Palestinian Central Bureau of Statistics (2000b) estimates that 3–4 percent of household income is spent on health care (including health insurance premiums) (Barnea and Husseini, 2002).

CHAPTER SIX

Strengthening Key Institutions, Policies, and Programs

For each of ten key areas, we present background information and our recommendations. We also briefly describe the effects of alternative scenarios. Our major recommendations are summarized in Table 6.1.

Health System Planning, Policy Development, and Policy Implementation

Background

During the period of Israeli administration (1967–1994), planning for the government health sector was led primarily by Israelis, with some Palestinian participation in policy formation and with Palestinian administrative support. Examples of joint policy development include the 1985 Adler Committee on health planning for the West Bank and standing committees such as the Child Health Committee in Gaza. Planning for UNRWA was mainly conducted at UNRWA headquarters in Vienna for all five areas of UNRWA activity (Syria, Lebanon, Jordan, West Bank, and Gaza), with some local Palestinian input. Government and UNRWA activities were coordinated to some degree, but many policies varied between these two sectors. The Israeli administration exercised some control over the NGO sector's infrastructure and programs. However, in many respects, NGOs explicitly aimed to compete with the government in the health sector for political reasons; coordination with the government was correspondingly low.

When Palestinian national health planning started in the years prior to the Oslo agreement, its leaders followed a process that was explicitly designed to be inclusive. The first national health plan called for the creation of a "health council" to oversee the health system, with the responsibility of developing strategic plans for future action, developing policy across both public and private health care programs, and monitoring and evaluating progress in meeting policy targets, among other functions. The plan called for this council, referred to as a "central authority," to involve all relevant

Table 6.1
Recommendations for Palestinian Health System Development

Area	Recommendation
Health system planning, policy development, and policy implementation	The Palestinian government should integrate health system planning and policy development more closely, with meaningful input from and coordination with all relevant governmental and nongovernmental stakeholders.
Health insurance and health care finance	The Palestinian government should develop viable and sustainable health insurance and health care financing systems.
Licensing and certification of health professionals	Palestinian standards for licensing and certifying all types of health professionals should be updated, standardized, and enforced.
Licensing and accreditation of health care facilities and services	Palestinian standards for licensing and accrediting health care facilities and services should be updated, standardized, and enforced.
Human resource development	Palestinian institutions should implement a human resource development strategy for the health professions to ensure an adequate supply of appropriately trained personnel for the Palestinian health system.
Health care quality improvement	A national strategy on health care quality improvement should be developed and implemented, with systematic evaluation of quality improvement projects and dissemination of those that succeed.
Policies on prescription drugs and medical devices	Policymakers should implement national strategies on the licensing, supply, and distribution of pharmaceuticals and medical devices to ensure a stable and adequate supply of safe and cost-effective products.
Health information systems	Palestinian policymakers should develop comprehensive, modern, and integrated health information systems.
Research	Palestinian policymakers should develop national strategies regarding public health, health services, clinical, and basic science research.
Programs for rapid improvement	The MOH should implement comprehensive programs to improve nutritional status, including food fortification, micronutrient supplementation for high-risk groups, and promotion of healthy dietary practices.
	The national immunization program should be updated, and the costs of purchasing and distributing vaccines should be explicitly covered by the government budget.
	The MOH and other stakeholders should expand the scope of available primary care services and expand access to comprehensive primary care.
	The MOH and other stakeholders should develop comprehensive strategies for addressing psychosocial needs, particularly those relating to the exposure of children to violence.

stakeholders in its activities, including "the private sector, the nonprofit sector, the university system, businesses, organized labor, and the voluntary sector," as well as local communities, and to ensure that these stakeholders participate in a meaningful way (Palestinian Council of Health, 1994).

In 1992, the Palestine Liberation Organization authorized the establishment of the Palestinian Council of Health, which completed the first Palestinian national health plan and acted as the national planning body until the MOH was established. This council included representatives from numerous NGOs, as well as private providers, academics, UNRWA, and other relevant stakeholders, all of which were involved in the council's activities.[1] Many council participants expected that this organization would serve as the "central authority" referred to in the first national health plan, once it became clear that responsibility for the Palestinian health system would be transferred to the PA under the Oslo agreement in 1994. As the MOH became established, however, many of the council's responsibilities—along with much of its staff—shifted to the new MOH. Although the council was not disbanded, it quickly stopped functioning as the national planning and coordination body for the health system.

As we have noted, national health planning has continued under the MOH, and the planning process has involved representatives from NGOs, the private sector, UNRWA, and the donor community. However, there is no systematic national process for ensuring that health system development is tailored to the goals articulated in the national health plan or other relevant planning documents. The MOH has had limited success exercising its managerial authority over the health system, and neither the MOH nor any other national institution provides effective overall coordination. Instead, there is a general lack of coordination in policy development and implementation across parts of the PA, between the West Bank and Gaza, and across the four major sectors of the health system (government, NGO, private, and UNRWA). Organizations across the four health sectors compete in an effort to advance their own priorities, rather than pursuing system-wide or national priorities; there is no consistent national process for reviewing new infrastructure projects to ensure that health infrastructure is developed efficiently; there are no modern standards for many key aspects of health system operation and minimal enforcement of the standards that do exist.[2] In addition, consumer input to the planning process has been limited.

In our view, the lack of coordination in policy development and implementation has limited progress toward achieving the health and health system targets specified in the national health plans, reduced the financial viability of the health care system, and

---

[1] Participation by Palestinian staff of the (Israeli) government health system was initially limited, for political reasons.

[2] In some ways, competition between NGOs and the government sector has intensified since 1994. Now, as under Israeli administration, some NGOs compete with the government sector, for ideological reasons and because of a scarcity of resources. Additionally, the MOH has competed with certain NGO activities, perhaps in an effort to establish authority over a health system in which several major NGOs were already well established when the MOH was created.

undermined public confidence in the government health system and possibly in the government generally. These conditions apply in some degree to nearly all aspects of the health system, including the development and operation of public health programs and clinical infrastructure, health care finance, and the pharmaceutical sector. One possible exception is human resources and health education, where the MOH and the Ministry of Education and Higher Education have recently established a body with authority to accredit any new health-related academic or vocational training program.

Recommendation: The Palestinian Government Should Integrate Health System Planning and Policy Development More Closely, with Meaningful Input from and Coordination with All Relevant Governmental and Nongovernmental Stakeholders

There are many ways to improve health system planning and coordination. However, effective planning and coordination processes are likely to share the features described below.

The planning and coordination processes should be implemented by a governmental authority. Nongovernmental stakeholders can help inform planning and the policymaking process, but they cannot independently develop national policy. National health planning, policymaking, and coordination across stakeholders should be led by a governmental body, with its responsibilities defined by legislation and/or regulation. Relevant areas of responsibility include

- overall responsibility for promoting the health of Palestinians
- establishment of national health priorities and targets
- financing of public health
- assurance of access to health care at the primary, secondary, and tertiary levels
- epidemiology and health status monitoring
- environmental quality and food and water safety
- safety and efficacy of pharmaceuticals and medical products
- maternal and child health
- control of communicable diseases
- control of noncommunicable diseases, injuries, and conditions
- legislation, licensing, and regulation of health care facilities and personnel (including educational standards)
- promotion of quality and equity in health care
- collection of national health accounting data and other data necessary for health system planning, policy development, and policy implementation.

It might seem that the most obvious entity for leading the planning process, and for coordinating across stakeholders, is the MOH. The MOH has led many of the health system planning efforts since 1994; it has considerable relevant expertise among its staff; and, at least in principle, the MOH already has responsibility for system-wide planning and coordination and at least some of the authority to carry it out. On the other hand, the MOH has had limited success to date in developing, implementing, and enforcing policy for the health system as a whole. For example, the MOH Health Sector Working Group—which includes the MOH, the Ministry of Planning, several international donors, the WHO, and other stakeholders—advises the MOH regarding policy development. But its decisions are not binding on the participating organizations, let alone on nonparticipating stakeholders. In addition, the MOH operates independently in Gaza and in the West Bank in many respects, even before the second intifada.

There are presumably many reasons for this, which will need to be addressed if an integrated planning process is to succeed. For instance, the MOH may have lacked the resources or expertise to implement effective planning and coordination at a national level; it may have lacked the necessary statutory authority; and/or it may have lacked the political will or ability to exercise such authority. Most interview participants favored the last of these explanations. In practice, the PA as a whole and most of its departments, including the MOH, have suffered from a weak level of authority over the sectors for which they are responsible; inefficient management practices; and autocratic, inconsistent, and nonparticipatory decisionmaking processes. The issue of Palestinian governance is discussed in more detail at the end of this chapter.

The MOH serves as a health care delivery system as well as a planning and regulatory body, creating the potential for conflicts of interest in the planning and policymaking process. It may therefore be beneficial to minimize the extent to which individuals or departments within the MOH have responsibility for both health care delivery and health system planning and policymaking. Options for distinguishing the two include creating a separate division within the MOH to be responsible for the government delivery system, creating an entirely separate agency with such responsibility, and privatizing health care delivery. Such options would need to be evaluated locally.

As an alternative method of broadening the policymaking process, national planning and coordination could be led by a new governmental body. The MOH would naturally play a significant role in this body, which would also include participants from the Ministries of Planning, Finance, and Education and Higher Education, and possibly other key players. To date, cooperation between the MOH and these other ministries regarding health policy has been limited, and effective cooperation may be more likely if all ministries jointly contribute to a new planning and coordination body.

Effective health planning and coordination also require appropriate oversight. The national planning and coordination body should ultimately be accountable to the prime minister; to the elected legislature, which defines the scope of the authority; and to the judicial system, which helps ensure that the body neither neglects nor exceeds its mandate. Many health systems have also developed formal processes for soliciting public input into planning and policymaking and an ombudsman process to help address consumer grievances.

Additional recommendations for strengthening the planning process are described below.

Health Planning Targets Should Reflect International Standards and Local Conditions. In many countries, and internationally, national targets for population health status, access to care, health care quality, and other indicators of health system performance play a vital role in guiding health system planning. Previous national health plans have included targets in some of these areas, framed largely in terms of local conditions. These targets should be revised and expanded on an ongoing basis, and they should reference—although not necessarily be identical to—international guidelines such as those developed by the WHO. Potential frames of reference for refining Palestinian targets include the WHO's Health for All in the 21st Century (online at http://www.who.int/archives/hfa/ [as of February 2004]) and the U.S. Healthy People 2010 targets (online at http://www.healthypeople.gov [as of May 2004]), in addition to data on health and health care in Palestine.

The Planning Process Should Be Inclusive. National health system planning should include meaningful participation by representatives from the NGO, private, and UNRWA sectors, in addition to government participants; from relevant professional associations (e.g., for physicians, nurses, pharmacists, etc.); from relevant academic institutions; from international donors; and especially from consumers and the community. Ensuring consumer representation in national planning bodies, making meetings open to the public, and including public hearings and a public comment period as part of policymaking are good strategies for promoting more comprehensive and effective consumer participation. Laws defining patients' rights can also strengthen the role of consumers in the planning and policymaking process; in Palestine, a draft patients' bill of rights was proposed by the Palestinian Council of Health, but no such policy has become law.

Formal participation by all stakeholders is likely to enhance the political and social legitimacy of the planning process and its outcomes, which in turn helps facilitate implementation of the plans.

Interview subjects expressed concern about the potential that the planning process might be "captured" by a small number of established stakeholders, or be dominated by specific personalities. Such issues are common to policymaking and regulatory bodies, and the planning process should be designed to reduce the chance of such outcomes.

Planning and Policymaking Should Be Integrated. The planning process should be comprehensive in scope and yield specific and measurable national targets for health status and health system development (in many ways, the previous national health plans have included such targets). These targets should guide policymaking for the health system.

In practice, the strategies for integrating planning and policymaking will differ for different stakeholders. In the government sector, the MOH and other ministries can be directed by statute or executive order to pursue such integration. It is important that health system budget allocations conform to and support national health development targets.

Government control over the policies of nongovernmental stakeholders is necessarily more limited; in particular, it is easier for the government to *prevent* donors or other organizations from implementing a particular project than to *compel* these organizations to implement a particular project. As a result, both regulatory oversight and positive incentives may be needed to increase integration with national plans. On the regulatory side, NGOs, private providers, or international donors can be required to seek approval for major capital investments, to ensure that infrastructure is developed in accordance with national plans; such an approval process should have established and transparent guidelines, and it should be binding. (This issue is further discussed under "Licensing and Accreditation of Health Care Facilities and Services" below.)

With respect to incentives, the MOH can use the coverage and payment rules of the government insurance programs to influence the scope and quality of service delivery in the private and NGO sectors; and it can increase commitment to the national health plans by including nongovernmental stakeholders in the planning process, as discussed above. Another possibility would be to establish an advisory panel of independent, international experts, which would advise the MOH and the national planning and coordination body and help provide support for policy decisions that are beneficial but may be unpopular.

Policy Implementation Should Be Strengthened. In the Palestinian health system, as in many other health systems, planning has frequently functioned better than policy implementation, and many of the aims of current and prior health plans have not been achieved. In our view, effective strategies for national health planning and coordination require that responsibility for implementing policy decisions be explicitly assigned to the appropriate stakeholders, with ongoing monitoring of implementation and appropriate incentives for successful performance. Subsequent recommendations in this book focus on the need to strengthen and maintain the skills of health system managers, evaluate new programs and policies, and collect comprehensive data about the health system.

Nearly all our interview participants expressed the view that the Palestinian government should *immediately* create a national planning and coordination authority with "teeth"—the power to ensure that health system policies and development projects conform to the national health plans. Although recognizing that such a body would influence and probably change how most health system stakeholders function, most interview participants considered its creation to be a necessary condition for addressing key problems in public health, health care access, health care quality, and financial viability of the health system. To the extent that opinions differed, they did so primarily with respect to the details of how such a planning body would be established and how it would function. However, even stakeholders in NGOs, the private sector, academic institutions, and international donor organizations agree that the planning body should be created under the auspices of the government, despite expressing concerns about the capabilities and the motivations of the MOH and the PA.

Effects of Restricted Domestic Mobility

Restricted mobility within Palestine would seriously inhibit essentially all aspects of health system planning, policy development, and policy implementation, as experience during the second intifada has shown. Since the start of the second intifada, the MOH has attempted few major development initiatives; those that have been attempted, such as a World Bank project on health information systems, have been delayed considerably; and coordination between MOH activities in the West Bank and Gaza has declined (from a level that was itself problematic). Continued restricted mobility would inhibit or prevent policymakers from meeting; inhibit or prevent oversight of health system functioning, including all types of data collection; and make implementation of new policies and programs more difficult and more costly.

Effects of Restricted International Access

Restricted international access would not necessarily inhibit the process of health system planning, policy development, and policy implementation, unless access by Palestinians to outside expertise and other resources is also restricted. However, it would affect the outcomes of the planning and policymaking process, by requiring that clinical and educational needs be met domestically. We discuss this further below.

Health Insurance and Health Care Finance

Background

During the period of Israeli administration, health insurance coverage was available primarily via the government health insurance plan; there was no private (commercial) health insurance, and informal insurance arrangements operated by NGOs were very limited. (Of course, the UNRWA health system functions as a health service benefit program for registered refugees.) Participation in the government plan was restricted to the groups who were required to enroll—i.e., government workers and Palestinians working in Israel. Under Israeli administration, the insurance program was priced to be largely self-funding, so that the annual premium corresponded to the average annual cost of covered services used by members. The Israeli administration had relatively strong control over the services offered in the government sector.

Nearly all Palestinians with health insurance obtain it through the MOH's insurance program. After 1994, some private health insurance was introduced, but these plans—which never enrolled more than 3 percent of the population—basically ended with the second intifada.

Although the government health plan is still closely based on the system that was introduced by Israel, the MOH has made several important changes. Perhaps the most fundamental change was to allow voluntary enrollment by individuals and households, and by employee groups that were not required to participate. At the same time, insurance premiums were reduced to promote enrollment.

The effects of such reductions on financial viability could have been positive if they had substantially increased enrollment by healthy people. However, allowing voluntary enrollment created the risk of adverse selection—in other words, that the people who chose to enroll were disproportionately sick. The risk of adverse selection was reinforced by the fact that people could enroll at almost any time, creating an incentive for healthy people to stay out of the system—and avoid paying insurance premiums—until they become sick or injured. As a particularly stark example, UNRWA pays to enroll people in the government insurance program when they are diagnosed with cancer; this is, in effect, an institutionalization of adverse selection.

Expansion of eligibility and reduction of premiums were intended to expand health insurance coverage and help reduce unmet need. In practice, however, the net effect of these changes was to increase the government system's liabilities more than it increased revenue, deepening the operating deficit that has existed since 1994 and threatening the survival of the system. Subsequent economic crises—and, of course, the decision after 2000 to waive premiums entirely for many people—have exacerbated the financial problems of the government insurance system.[3]

In contrast to the enrollment rules and premiums, the benefit structure of the government health plan has changed very little over time. Members face no cost sharing for outpatient office visits, but co-payments are required for diagnostic services such as laboratory tests and imaging. Many health insurance plans in other countries work in exactly the opposite fashion, the rationale being that patients have relatively strong control over the decision to see the doctor, but relatively weak control over the diagnostic services the doctor prescribes. The government plan also requires co-payments for prescription drugs but not for inpatient care with appropriate referral; both are features that have been widely adopted in foreign health insurance plans. Moreover, the "gatekeeping" aspect of the referral system for inpatient care is not always applied rigorously, and patients who seek such a referral are generally able to receive one.

The government health system does not include systematic utilization review for outpatient care, such as requiring primary care referral for specialty care. We recognize that the potential effect of primary care gatekeeping is likely to be muted, at least in the short run, by the current shortage of specialists in many clinical areas. Patients in the government health sector (and in UNRWA) have little ability to choose providers, except by opting to receive care in a different sector.

The government plan covers care only from government providers, unless patients are specifically referred to private or NGO providers, or to providers abroad, for care that cannot be provided in the government sector. The reliance on government services has both clinical and financial motivations. The former reflect concerns about incon-

---

[3] We note that even waiving the health insurance premiums has not lead to universal insurance coverage, one stated goal of the national health plans. Coverage is estimated to be around 80 percent at the time of this writing, apparently because not everyone who is eligible has actually enrolled. When premiums were required, health insurance coverage peaked at 55 percent of households, including families whose insurance coverage was sponsored by the government under the hardship program—also far short of universal coverage.

sistent quality and lack of government oversight in the private and NGO sectors. The latter reflect a desire to avoid the open-ended liabilities that might arise from paying NGO and private providers on a fee-for-service basis, while government providers are salaried. In practice, however, the government sector has been unable to meet the demand for its services, particularly following the large increase in insurance enrollment since premiums were waived. At the same time, the MOH lacks the economic resources—and the statutory authority—to shift some of this excess demand to the private or NGO sectors. The result has been considerable overcrowding of government facilities and a perceived decline in quality of care—while simultaneously some private and NGO facilities are underutilized.

Several other factors affect care in the government sector. For instance, as is true in many developing areas, the government salary structure serves as an incentive for public providers to maintain private practices on the side, by choice or out of economic necessity. This dual role may distract public providers from the responsibilities of their government positions and create other conflicts of interest. The relatively centralized management structure of the public sector offers few positive incentives to facility administrators and individual clinicians to provide health care efficiently. For example, senior hospital staff are generally appointed by the MOH rather than by the hospital director. Hospital managers are not provided with specific budgets for operating their facilities, and accountability by hospital managers for the use of pharmaceuticals and other consumables in their facilities is often weak. At the same time, all health care sectors lack modern health information systems, particularly relating to hospital discharge data and other indicators of health system performance. This makes it very difficult to implement an efficient system of local accountability, since it inhibits planning and evaluation of facility performance.

Overall, the government health sector has operated at a deficit since its inception in 1994. Government liabilities have considerably exceeded the sum of health insurance premiums and general tax revenues allocated to the health sector. Communication between the MOH and the Ministry of Finance (which determines or at least administers budget allocations) is poor, and there have been periods of crisis (e.g., in 1997) when the Ministry of Finance did not allocate the expected budget to the MOH. The PA effectively doubled enrollment in the government health insurance system when it recently waived premiums, but these increased liabilities were not reflected in the budget planning process. Indeed, it appears that the government did not explicitly account for the liabilities it incurred when it lowered insurance premiums in the mid-1990s to promote enrollment in the government program.

System-wide, a substantial part of the cost of health care services has been borne by patients in the form of out-of-pocket spending. However, there is a perception of considerable unmet need for health care in Palestine—even while all sectors of the health system (except perhaps the private sector) have received considerable external subsidies. The operating budget of the MOH has been directly supported by foreign donors, and indirectly supported by the high volume of services provided in other sectors to patients who are formally entitled to receive the care in the government sector. Similarly, with the exception of patient cost sharing, the entire UNRWA sector is externally financed by design (UNRWA also subsidizes the government system, to the extent that it provides services that patients would otherwise be entitled to receive from the government system). Finally, most NGOs subsidize the care they provide with funding from local and foreign sources.[4]

Recommendation: The Palestinian Government Should Develop Viable and Sustainable Health Insurance and Health Care Financing Systems

Addressing these complex issues is difficult in any health care system. However, successful policies are likely to include some common features, as described below.

The Planning Target Should Be Universal Health Coverage. Most health systems that are regarded as "successful," in the sense intended by our mandate, have achieved universal—or close to universal—health insurance coverage. The previous national health plans have included the goal of universal health insurance coverage in Palestine. We think maintenance of this goal and good faith efforts to achieve it are important for social and political reasons—a view supported by all our interview participants.

Interview participants (and the policy literature) suggested a range of possible strategies, without any obvious consensus. Some participants thought that achieving this goal needs to be deferred for the foreseeable future and favored continuing the current government system and its provision for voluntary enrollment. Others favored mandatory and universal participation in a national insurance program but differed in how comprehensive the benefits of such a program should be. For instance, one option might be to provide a "core" benefit, available to everybody, that covers a basic set of services (e.g., public health, preventive care, and basic curative services). People could supplement this core benefit, if they chose, by purchasing more comprehensive private coverage. Opinions also differed on the appropriate role for government versus private insurance. As is always the case in insurance, the risk-pooling benefits of universal government coverage are likely to trade off against the restricted choice and potentially poor quality that arise in such a system. In our view, these issues need to be resolved locally.

Demand-Side Incentives for Efficient Health Care Use Should Be Improved. We assume that the government insurance program will be maintained in the future, in some form. However, its benefit structure should be updated to encourage both patients and providers to use care more efficiently. On the demand side, available evidence from developed and developing countries suggests that modest levels of patient cost sharing for many types of health care services help control health care costs without adversely affecting health outcomes (appropriate co-payment levels would be determined locally).Similarly, there is evidence that utilization review and care management tech-

---

[4] We note that market-based health reform strategies often seek to promote competition, particularly on the basis of cost and quality. One implication of the significant level of subsidies in the Palestinian health system is that the competition across and within sectors of this stystem is not necessarily market based. In particular, UNRWA, NGOs, and international donors are not simply making "investments" in the business sense.

niques can help control costs and/or improve outcomes, particularly among patients with chronic medical conditions (such as diabetes, asthma, hypertension, and heart disease) that commonly involve acute complications and hospitalization. Updated cost sharing and utilization review mechanisms should be based on international evidence and local economic circumstances.

Government policies currently provide universal entitlement to preventive health services without patient cost sharing. In general, the scope of preventive services is relatively comprehensive for children, particularly up to age three. However, there is considerable room to expand the scope of such services, for both children and—perhaps especially—adults. As we discuss further below, government strategies regarding nutritional status require updating and expansion, particularly for high-risk groups. (The MOH released a new national nutrition strategy in July 2003; it is too early to know what its effects will be.) With respect to the general adult population, available epidemiological evidence suggests high and increasing prevalence of chronic diseases—notably diabetes, hypertension, and heart disease—for which primary and secondary prevention efforts can be quite effective. Although these conditions are associated with considerable expenditure on tertiary care, health education and prevention efforts for these conditions are relatively underdeveloped. Increased prevention efforts in these and other areas have the potential to reduce total health care costs.

Supply-Side Incentives for Efficient Health Care Use Should Be Improved. The MOH (or the national health planning authority) should improve incentives for the efficient supply of health services, particularly in the government sector. These improvements should include better management practices for government health facilities—e.g., by implementing formal budgeting processes, holding facility managers accountable for clinical and financial performance, and providing local staff with greater authority and autonomy. Other possible steps include giving individual providers incentives to meet specific evidence-based performance benchmarks and minimizing conflicts of interest between government providers' public and private practices. We note that performance incentives do not necessarily have to be monetary; other possible incentives include peer recognition, training or research support, and additional vacation time.

Effective implementation of such strategies is likely to require improved information systems, which we discuss in greater detail under "Health Information Systems" below.

Coverage Rules for Tertiary Care Referrals Should Be Specific, Publicized, and Implemented Consistently. Tertiary care capabilities in Palestine are currently limited. Additional tertiary care capabilities, including development and operation, are expensive, and the cost to the MOH of referring patients for treatment abroad—whether to Israel, neighboring countries such as Jordan or Egypt, or to Europe—is also considerable. Given scarce resources, the MOH has worked to reduce the rate of such referrals by expanding local capacity and by making referral criteria more restrictive. In general, such efforts are likely to be beneficial for the health system overall. However, both strategies should be implemented systematically and transparently.

Strategies for expanding local capacity should reflect both the relative cost and the relative quality of treatment abroad. In particular, the Palestinian population is relatively small, and there are likely to be many conditions for which the national incidence rate will be below the minimum volume necessary to sustain a clinically successful treatment program. It may be both clinically and economically efficient to develop tertiary care "centers of excellence," focusing on high-impact conditions that are also relatively prevalent. In any case, development of tertiary care facilities should conform to the strategies and targets determined by the national health planning process.

Referrals for care abroad could also be more systematic and cost-effective. The MOH is likely to benefit from negotiating bilateral agreements with foreign countries or institutions regarding referral of Palestinian patients. The MOH has already negotiated some agreements with foreign institutions, but our understanding is that these agreements do not specify the rates that the MOH will be charged for care. Future agreements should include rate schedules for specific types of care.

Israel is one obvious place to refer Palestinian patients, for reasons of geography and of health system capacity and quality. Indeed, the MOH has referred many patients to Israeli institutions since 1994 and continues to do so. Several interview participants pointed out, however, that Israeli institutions charge the MOH the equivalent of "tourist" rates for Palestinian referrals; i.e., higher rates than these institutions charge for treating the members of Israeli health insurance plans. Although this may reflect economic realities, most notably the risk of nonpayment or incomplete payment, we recommend that the referral terms be renegotiated to be more favorable to Palestinian patients. In our view, this would benefit all parties.

Criteria for determining whether patients are referred outside the government health system, domestically or abroad, should be detailed, transparent, and applied consistently.

Policymakers Should Consider Covering Care in the Private and NGO Sectors. As described above, the government health insurance program does not generally cover services provided outside the government health sector. At the same time, many government facilities are already operating at the limits of their capacity, and they are certainly not adequate for meeting the needs of the entire population. The MOH will therefore need to expand the government health sector significantly, and/or expand the role of private and NGO providers under the government insurance program, as it works toward achieving the national goal of comprehensive universal health insurance coverage.

Private and NGO providers currently represent a substantial part of health system capacity (see Table 5.3 in Chapter Five). To the extent that these providers meet appropriate criteria regarding quality and costs, it is likely to be more efficient for the MOH to purchase care from them than to replace them. In particular, policymakers should avoid devoting scarce development resources to building redundant capacity—i.e., building or expanding government capacity in areas where private and NGO capacity is available and adequate. We recommend against having the government sector provide all care, because such a monopoly might weaken incentives for quality and efficiency.

Such expansion may be more feasible and appropriate in the context of improved national planning, policy development, and policy implementation, as discussed above; strengthened national licensing and certification standards (discussed further below under "Licensing and Certification of Health Professionals" and "Licensing and Accreditation of Health Care Facilities and Services"); transparency in financial accounting for all stakeholders; and cost-control mechanisms for care in the private/NGO sectors, such as standardized fee schedules for specific health services, primary care gatekeeping, and preauthorization requirements for care from nongovernment providers. Particularly in the context of such developments, the MOH could use inclusion in the government health benefit as an incentive to private and NGO providers to promote quality and efficiency.

Policymakers Should Develop Contingency Plans Regarding East Jerusalem. As we have described, Israel currently has responsibility for the health system in East Jerusalem. Residents of East Jerusalem are covered by the compulsory Israeli national health insurance program and are thus enrolled in one of the four Israeli "sick" funds that cover primary, secondary, and tertiary care. Health care providers and facilities in this system are governed by Israeli protocols.

This book would be incomplete without some consideration of the possibility that responsibility for the health system of East Jerusalem will shift to the government of a future independent Palestinian state. In particular, patterns of health and health care use and costs in East Jerusalem are currently closer to Israeli standards than to those in Palestine. On the one hand, without substantial outside subsidies, the Palestinian health system will certainly lack the resources to maintain current levels of provider reimbursement and overall spending for Palestinians in East Jerusalem. On the other hand, significant reductions in reimbursement levels and overall spending in East Jerusalem are likely to cause considerable harm to its health care infrastructure. The MOH and other relevant stakeholders (e.g., other ministries, health care providers in East Jerusalem, the Israeli Ministry of Health, and international donors) should consider specific strategies for incorporating the health system of East Jerusalem into the broader Palestinian health system.

Several interview participants raised the possibility that net contributions by Palestinian residents of East Jerusalem to the Israeli health insurance programs have been positive (i.e., contributions have exceeded the cost of health care use). This could arise, for instance, for groups that are younger than the population average. They argued that, if this were true, Palestinians who had historically been covered by Israeli insurance have an entitlement to continued participation in the Israeli system. The rationale is that national social insurance involves risk sharing between healthy and unhealthy people not just at a point in time, but over time as well (i.e., as people age, they use more health care for age-associated reasons). We did not evaluate this issue here.

The Palestinian Government Should Work with Other Stakeholders, Particularly International Donors, to Establish Stable and Adequate Health System Funding. Since 1994, local resources have not been sufficient to sustain the Palestinian health system at current levels, which in any case do not meet our mandate of a truly successful Palestinian health system. Some of the policy options described above have the potential to reduce costs and/or increase efficiency, and thus to promote financial viability. Nevertheless, we believe that achieving a successful Palestinian health system will require considerable outside resources for the foreseeable future. (We discuss levels of external support in Chapter Eight.) Given the current and likely future role of the government sector, many of these resources will need to be directed to the government health system for the overall health system to function successfully.

However, as prior analyses of the Palestinian health system have emphasized, such an approach conflicts directly with the policies and priorities of many international donors, who strongly favor channeling resources through NGOs rather than through government entities, and who also favor making capital investments rather than supporting operating budgets. In recognition of the limitations of these strategies, in July 2003, the U.S. government authorized $20 million of direct support to the PA, the first such payment since the PA was established.[5] Additional direct cooperation between the Palestinian government and international donors is needed to facilitate successful future health system development and operation.

Effects of Restricted Domestic Mobility

Health insurance benefits should reflect patients' abilities to reach appropriate health care facilities. For instance, if patients cannot travel to distant government facilities, it may be necessary for the government health benefit to cover care in the NGO and private sectors on more than the current exceptional basis. If mobility is restricted, however, even such expanded coverage will leave many people with inadequate access to care, particularly secondary and tertiary care in rural areas. We discuss the implications of restricted mobility on access to care and health infrastructure development further below under "Licensing and Accreditation of Health Care Facilities and Services."

Restricted domestic mobility would also significantly impair health system management. While it would necessarily increase the authority of local managers—something we recommend, in principle—it would inhibit national systems of oversight and accountability. On a related issue, restricted mobility would inhibit or prevent the collection of most types of health system data; we discuss this further below under "Health Information Systems."

---

[5] Of this total, $11 million were slated for specific infrastructure projects, including the repair of municipal water and sewage systems; road repair and reconstruction; repair of electrical distribution lines; and rehabilitation of municipal schools, clinics, courthouses, and other public buildings. Up to $9 million were intended to ensure the continued provision of electric, water, and sewage utility services.

More generally, restricted mobility is likely to limit the economic viability of a Palestinian state and correspondingly reduce the resources available for health system development. In principle, this could be offset by additional external resources. However, the availability of certain sources of funding, particularly private investment, is likely to be positively related to the economic viability of the state.

Effects of Restricted International Access

Health insurance policies regarding referrals for care abroad will obviously depend on whether and to where such referrals are possible.

On a related issue, if the Israeli labor market is open to Palestinian workers to any significant degree, we recommend that the Palestinian health planning authority (or the MOH in its absence), the Israeli Ministry of Health, and other relevant organizations develop coordinated policies regarding health insurance coverage and health care for Palestinians working in Israel.

Licensing and Certification of Health Professionals

Background

According to the second national health plan, there are approximately 2,000 physicians in Palestine. Since the only Palestinian medical school, at Al-Quds University, was established in 1994 and graduated its first class in 2001, essentially all practicing physicians in Palestine were trained elsewhere.[6] Although we know of no systematic inventory of where physicians practicing in Palestine were trained, it is clear that their training has varied widely and may be incomplete and out-of-date in many cases. For instance, many Soviet medical graduates who emigrated to Israel in the 1990s required additional training before qualifying for an Israeli medical license, suggesting that the many Palestinian graduates of Soviet medical schools might also require additional training to meet appropriate practice standards.

Historically, and today, Palestinian physicians must receive a license to practice. In both the West Bank and Gaza, candidates are required to pass examinations in order to be licensed, although procedures differ in these two areas. The West Bank's licensing protocols are modeled on those in Jordan, while Gaza's protocols are modeled on those in Egypt. However, these licensing criteria have not been consistently applied since the PA assumed responsibility for health care in 1994; as a result, some physicians received licenses without meeting the minimum criteria. Moreover, physicians and other health professionals are licensed for life; and they are not required to participate in continuing education to maintain their skills, nor to demonstrate continued proficiency as a condition of maintaining their medical license.

---

[6] Indeed, a number of Al-Quds medical graduates are currently receiving postgraduate training abroad.

As a related issue, the institutions controlling subspecialty certification are weak or absent. Subspecialty certification is particularly problematic in Gaza, partly because Egyptian protocols regarding subspecialty training are relatively weak and partly because there have been few attempts to enforce existing standards. As a result, many physicians in Gaza represent themselves as subspecialists of various types without having completed adequate subspecialty training.

To our knowledge, no systematic and ongoing program of continuing medical education (CME) currently exists in Palestine; hence, even providers who would voluntarily participate in CME may have difficulty doing so. Although many training programs have been offered over the past decade, sponsored by many different organizations, they have typically been conducted once or twice, not on a systematic, ongoing basis to successive cohorts of providers. We also know of no standard processes for suspending or revoking a medical license in case of malpractice or professional misconduct, or for individual or class-action lawsuits in such cases.

In our interviews, several people proposed reasons why continuing education has not been established despite widespread consensus regarding its importance. These included the economic cost of participating in training and possible provider reluctance to let their patients know that they were receiving continuing education (e.g., because this might undermine patients' confidence).

With few exceptions, conditions are similar for nurses, pharmacists, and other health professionals: Initial training often needs to be improved; standards of licensing are weak and/or inconsistently enforced; and licenses are valid for life, without any requirement to participate in continuing education programs. As is the case with physicians, no institutionalized CME programs are available for nurses, pharmacists, and other health professionals on even a voluntary basis.

Information from published reports and our interview stakeholders supports the view that weak licensing requirements and the lack of CME combine to reduce quality of care, in some cases to unacceptably low levels. Moreover, as is true in many countries, Palestinian consumers have difficulty distinguishing high-quality providers from those who are unqualified—a difficulty compounded by the fact that existing licensing standards are inconsistently applied and that there are no systematic legal remedies for addressing acute problems.

Recommendation: Palestinian Standards for Licensing and Certifying All Types of Health Professionals Should Be Updated, Standardized, and Enforced

Effective licensing and certification programs are likely to share some common features, as described below.

Licensing and Certification Standards Should Be Valid Measures of Providers' Qualifications. The purpose of these standards is to ensure that all licensed providers have demonstrated the knowledge and skill to provide effective care. It obviously follows from this that licensing and certification standards should be valid measures of this knowledge and skill—both at the time of initial licensing and over time.

In principle, licensing exams and subspecialty certification criteria could be developed locally, based on international standards; or exams and criteria from elsewhere could be used directly (e.g., those from Jordan, which are already used in the West Bank). Given the limited size of the Palestinian health system, particularly in subspecialty fields, we recommend the latter.[7]

The Licensing and Certification Processes Should Be Implemented with Governmental Authority. In most health systems, licensing of physicians, nurses, pharmacists, and other health professionals is a government function. In Palestine, this function would most naturally be implemented by the MOH, but it could also be implemented by an independent organization or by another body with MOH oversight. Practices vary with regard to subspecialty certification, which is sometimes implemented by government and sometimes by an independent body under government authority. The appropriate model for Palestine should be determined locally.

In any case, licensing and certification standards should have the force of law— i.e., practicing without a license, or violating the terms of the license, should lead to civil and/or criminal sanctions. In addition, there should be established procedures for suspending or revoking licenses in the case of malpractice or misconduct.

Licensing and Certification Standards Should Apply to All Palestinian Providers. A single set of standards for the West Bank and Gaza and for all sectors of the health system would minimize the cost of these programs and maximize their benefit for consumers. Different standards add complexity and cost, impose unnecessary constraints on practice patterns if providers are licensed in one area or sector but not another, and confuse consumers.

Adequate Levels of Accredited Continuing Education Should Be a Condition of Maintaining the License/Certification. Effective licensing and certification standards require the availability of high-quality continuing education programs for all types of health professionals. These programs can be implemented by the MOH, NGOs, academic institutions, and others; and by domestic or international organizations.[8] However, all continuing education programs should be relevant to local conditions, and they should be accredited. We discuss accreditation of training programs in detail below.

One factor that has inhibited the development of continuing medical education in Palestine is the economic burden CME imposes on providers. Such education could

---

[7] For instance, in the United States, subspecialty certification standards are developed by professional organizations for each subspecialty. In Palestine, however, the total number of subspecialists in many fields is too small to support an effective professional association for each field.

[8] In our interviews, various people reported that the organizations they represented were interested in developing and offering ongoing CME programs if the policies of the MOH and the relevant professional associations supported such training.

be required and uncompensated (in effect, a "cost of doing business"). Alternatively, providers could receive some compensation for participation, at least initially. The issue of compensation is presumably most acute for nonsalaried providers, in the NGO and private sectors (government and UNRWA providers are generally salaried). This issue can best be resolved locally as part of the policymaking and implementation process.

Palestinian organizations, like those in other countries, have begun to use distance learning methods for training in health and other areas. Expanded use of such methods may facilitate the quality of continuing programs (e.g., by providing easier access to outside experts) and reduce their costs.

The Licensing and Certification Standards Should Include Explicit Policies Regarding Current—and Potentially Underqualified—Providers. Any time that new licensing standards are introduced, there is a question of how these standards will affect providers who were licensed using prior standards. Palestinian policymakers will need to determine whether and how existing providers should be required to meet whatever new licensing requirements are developed, whether they should be permitted to relicense on a voluntary basis, or whether they should be totally or partially exempted under a "grandfather clause." If existing providers are not required to comply with new standards, an alternative might be to develop conventions for naming the new credentials that could be used only by providers who meet the new standards.

Of these options, mandatory relicensing is likely to have the biggest effect on improving providers' knowledge, and consumers would need to recognize only a single licensing standard. However, it may be politically difficult to implement, involve relatively high training costs, and risk producing a shortage of providers (e.g., if many existing providers are unable or unwilling to qualify). Voluntary relicensing is likely to be easier to implement than a mandatory program; and the effects of such a program could be enhanced through consumer education about the new standards as a signal of provider quality, and/or through financial incentives from the MOH and other payers for relicensing. These issues should be resolved locally.

We note that many of the issues covered in this subsection were examined in greater detail in the *National Plan for Human Resource Development and Education in Health.* In general, we consider the goals and strategies outlined in that plan to remain relevant, and we refer readers to that report for additional details (Welfare Association, PA, and Ministry of Higher Education, 2001a–f).[9]

Effects of Restricted Domestic Mobility

Limited population mobility would make it difficult to implement and enforce appropriate standards of licensing and certification. By inhibiting access for both faculty and students, it would also prevent the development and implementation of high-quality continuing education programs. These effects could be mitigated with additional fi-

---

[9] Dr. Afifi, one of the authors of this book, was overall project coordinator for the development of the *National Plan for Human Resource Development and Education in Health.*

nancial resources to pay for operating local-area licensing, certification, and training. However, doing so would be costly, and it is unlikely that enough appropriate personnel would be available to implement these programs in all areas.

Effects of Restricted International Access

Licensing, certification, and continuing education activities are generally implemented domestically. However, restricted access could limit access by Palestinians to outside expertise and other resources, and thus inhibit the development and implementation of effective licensing and certification programs.

Licensing and Accreditation of Health Care Facilities and Services

Background

As with the process for licensing health professionals, the processes for licensing and accrediting health care facilities and services in Palestine should be strengthened. In general, the MOH has authority to review and approve new infrastructure development projects that are proposed for the health system and also to set standards for the operation of existing facilities and services. However, the MOH has exercised this authority in a very limited fashion. Current standards for licensing new projects and for reviewing existing facilities and programs are relatively weak, and they are inconsistently applied and enforced. Moreover, many practices continue to differ between the West Bank and Gaza.

As a result, new infrastructure projects do not always conform to the health development targets of the national health plans, nor to any other coordinated national strategy; and low-quality facilities and services are allowed to operate, with little pressure to improve. For example, the European Hospital in Gaza was built despite the fact that it did not conform to national development strategies for inpatient care. Following its completion in 1997, it remained unused for more than three years because the MOH lacked the money and staff to operate it.

Many types of health services fail to meet consistent standards. For example, the law prohibiting pharmacists from dispensing medication to patients without a physician's prescription is rarely enforced. As another example, an increasing number of ambulance services operating in Palestine do not meet national (or other internationally accepted) standards for training, equipment, and overall quality. The Palestine Red Crescent Society (PRCS) has statutory authority to set standards for ambulance services. However, to be effective, these standards must be enforced by the government, which has generally not happened. PRCS has offered to provide equipment and supplies to ambulance services that voluntarily conform to the PRCS national standards, but this strategy has also not generally led to compliance. Similarly, the PRCS has developed practice guidelines for prehospital emergency care, while the MOH and other stakeholders are currently developing a parallel set of standards.

A somewhat related issue is the long-run integration and operation of the new infrastructure that has been developed in the context of the second intifada and the associated geographic closures. Although the local facilities developed since 2000 have helped to increase access to health care under conditions of closure, under conditions of peace many of these facilities may not be clinically effective or economically efficient because of low patient volume. If free travel is allowed in a future independent Palestinian state, policymakers will need to determine how (or whether) to integrate these new facilities into the national health system.

Recommendation: Palestinian Standards for Licensing and Accrediting Health Care Facilities and Services Should Be Updated, Standardized, and Enforced

Successful licensing and accreditation systems are likely to include some common features, as described below.

New Infrastructure Development Should Be Consistent with National Strategies and Targets. To promote efficient infrastructure development, many health systems require that new health system infrastructure projects be licensed. To be successful, such a process should have specific and transparent guidelines, such as requiring that new infrastructure projects be consistent with national development targets. Licensing requirements should be binding, regardless of funding source or sponsoring organization. As discussed above, this process would fall under the national health planning authority.

The Licensing and Certification Processes Should Be Implemented with Governmental Authority. As described under licensing of health professionals, this function can be carried out directly by the government, or by an independent body under government authority.

The Licenses/Accreditation of Facilities and Programs Should Be Reevaluated Periodically. As with health care providers, a policy of licensing facilities and programs "for life" is unlikely to maximize their effectiveness and efficiency. Facilities and programs should therefore be reevaluated periodically. Every effort should be made to strengthen those that do not meet current standards; in extreme cases, however, the authority should exist to close facilities and programs temporarily. Evaluation standards should be specific, transparent, and national; and they should be applied consistently to government, private, NGO, and UNRWA facilities and programs. Evaluation of government and UNRWA facilities by an independent body may help reduce conflict of interest.

Licensing and Accreditation Standards Should Be Valid Measures of Facility and Program Performance. The purpose of these standards is to ensure that all approved facilities and programs are providing care that is adequately effective and efficient. The standards should be valid measures of such performance.

The Government Health System and Other Payers Should Consider Explicit Incentives to Promote Quality. Many health systems are using, or are considering the use of, financial incentives for health care facilities and programs that meet certain performance benchmarks. Such strategies may complement national licensing and accreditation standards, which are generally designed to ensure that institutions meet a minimum threshold of quality. We discuss these and other strategies further under "Health Care Quality Improvement" below.

Effects of Restricted Domestic Mobility

Limited population mobility would make it difficult to implement and enforce appropriate standards of licensing and accreditation. As discussed above, it would also require significantly different health infrastructure development strategies. In particular, it would require much greater emphasis on local delivery of clinical services. However, it would be difficult or impossible to provide all needed services in all areas, particularly secondary and tertiary services; moreover, the costs associated with developing many local facilities would be higher than that of a system based on fewer referral centers, and clinical quality is likely to be lower because of low patient volume.

Even assuming contiguous Palestinian territory in the West Bank and unrestricted access to East Jerusalem, the Palestinian health system is likely to face the challenge of a physically separate Gaza. If so, national health planners will need to determine whether it is more efficient to develop separate secondary and tertiary care capabilities in Gaza and the West Bank, versus investing in patient transport systems, international referral, or other strategies. In any case, we recommend that Palestinian health planners focus on developing national institutions with common standards and programs across all Palestinian territories.

Effects of Restricted International Access

Licensing and accreditation are generally implemented domestically. However, restricted international access for patients could affect strategies for infrastructure development. Given the size of the Palestinian population and the current capabilities of its health system, a strategy of domestic provision of all types of health care—including secondary and tertiary services—is unlikely to be economically or clinically efficient. Developing an infrastructure to deliver all types of care domestically (rather than referring some patients to foreign institutions for specialty care) is likely to result in higher costs and lower quality.

Human Resource Development

Background

Along with licensing and certification procedures, Palestinian educational programs need to be strengthened for all types of health professionals, including clinicians, pharmacists, health system administrators, public health workers, research and evaluation staff, and other relevant personnel. In many of these fields, the supply of appropriately trained professionals for the Palestinian health system is currently inadequate.

As noted above, there is one medical school in Palestine, which currently admits 40–50 new undergraduate students per year. The medical training program needs to be strengthened academically to meet international standards, with respect to both basic science and clinical education. Although some internship posts are available in Palestinian institutions and more are being developed, postgraduate medical training in Palestine is currently very limited. Our interview participants noted that Palestinian medical graduates must go abroad to receive suitable subspecialty training in nearly all fields, including primary care subspecialties such as general internal medicine and family practice.

Overall, the number of physicians per capita generally conforms to targets set in the national health plans. However, the supply of highly qualified physicians is limited, particularly in many medical subspecialties. Specific areas of shortage mentioned by interview participants included psychology, psychiatry (particularly child psychiatry), neurology, and oncology (particularly radiation oncology), among others.

There are also two dental schools in Palestine, which were established more recently than the medical school. Training programs in other clinical areas, including nursing, pharmacy, midwifery, medical social work, and psychology, were established before the medical school. Together, the capacities of these programs come closer to meeting Palestinian national needs in their respective areas than does the medical school. However, there is a shortage of qualified professionals in many areas, including dentistry, nursing, midwifery, and psychosocial medicine, and there may be some degree of excess in pharmacy (or at least in the current number of private pharmacies).[10] Moreover, there was widespread consensus among those we interviewed that the quality of all types of training programs needed to be improved.

We were unable to assess the supply and quality of training of other health professionals, such as administrators, public health workers, and research and evaluation staff. However, it is likely that these areas also require strengthening. We emphasize the importance of focusing on training in each of these areas as part of any national human resource development program in health, particularly since these areas are often underemphasized relative to training programs for clinicians.

Finally, successful human resource development for the Palestinian health system is likely to require improved salary and working conditions, particularly in the government sector. Interview participants who were *not* themselves public employees consistently commented on the acute lack of resources in the public sector for recruiting and retaining highly qualified staff. Limited resources, along with weak civil service institutions and the perceived lack of a stable career path for public health sector employees, may be causing some qualified staff to move from the government sector to the private sector, to NGOs (particularly those with international funding, some of which offer salaries that vastly exceed the government pay scale), or abroad. A related problem suggested by our nongovernmental interview participants is that the organi-

---

[10] Validating these perceptions was outside the scope of our analysis.

zational structure of the MOH, particularly the fragmentation of responsibility across departments, negatively affects employee performance and willingness to remain in the public sector.

Recommendation: Palestinian Institutions Should Implement a Human Resource Development Strategy for the Health Professions to Ensure an Adequate Supply of Appropriately Trained Personnel for the Palestinian Health System

Successful strategies for achieving this goal are likely to include a number of features, as described below.

Existing Educational Institutions and Programs Should Be Accredited, Using Appropriate International Standards. Many countries have implemented minimum accreditation standards that medical, dental, and nursing schools and other educational institutions and programs must meet for their programs to be allowed to operate and for their graduates to be eligible for professional licensing and certification. These accreditation standards are implemented with government authority, but they can be defined and assessed by governmental or nongovernmental organizations.

In Palestine, the Ministry of Education and Higher Education has responsibility for authorizing the establishment of new educational programs and for monitoring existing programs. However, health education programs have not consistently been held to high standards of quality, neither at the time they were established nor over time. This has a number of implications, including the likelihood that graduates' initial training may be inadequate and that graduates may have limited access to further training—particularly abroad—because their initial degrees do not meet international standards.

Addressing shortcomings in educational quality will require development and application of appropriate accreditation standards. These standards should be based on appropriate international models. International standards are likely to be useful in their own right, and adherence to international standards facilitates educational exchange for undergraduate and graduate training.[11]

We expect that many educational programs will require strengthening to meet accreditation standards. Strengthening domestic training programs will require a national investment strategy to recruit and retain suitable faculty and to build, maintain, and operate the infrastructure necessary to support training. Programs that repeatedly fail to meet accreditation criteria should be closed until the standards are met.

Under conditions of peace, Israel is likely to be a valuable source of technical assistance, particularly regarding faculty development and research. Israeli institutions have played this role successfully in the past, and Israeli stakeholders consistently reported that their institutions would be willing to do so in the future, circumstances and resources permitting.

---

[11] In the absence of a suitable Palestinian accreditation program, the medical school at Al-Quds University has directly pursued accreditation by British and U.S. institutions. It is also currently pursuing accreditation by Israel; because of the location of the medical school, Israeli policy requires such accreditation.

The MOH and the Ministry of Education and Higher Education have recently established a body that must authorize any new health-related academic or vocational training program in health. This approach is consistent with the recommendations outlined in this book. This body is relatively new, so there has not yet been an opportunity to evaluate its performance systematically.

Existing Health Education Programs Should Meet Minimum Accreditation Standards Before New Programs Are Established. New programs are likely to compete with existing programs for scarce human, physical, and financial resources, risking a reduction in overall quality and limited success in achieving the programs' objectives. Perhaps the most salient example of this is the medical school at Al-Quds University, which was opened in 1994 without its own teaching and laboratory facilities, equipment, library, complete curriculum, or adequate faculty and staff. Indeed, the school was established despite a recommendation by the Palestine Council on Higher Education (later the Ministry of Higher Education, and now the Ministry of Education and Higher Education), based on a feasibility study and internal workshop, that the opening of a Palestinian medical school be delayed. In our view, the medical school has had limited success in achieving the goals for which it was established, which included improvement of health care quality, CME, and clinical research in Palestine. Whether it will achieve the goal of producing competent physicians to serve the Palestinian population is still unknown because the first cohorts of graduates have not yet completed their training.

It may be beneficial to delay the establishment of new degree-granting educational programs in health until the corresponding existing programs have been evaluated by the Ministry of Education and Higher Education, and after strategies are in place to strengthen these existing programs in accordance with appropriate accreditation standards. (By "corresponding" existing programs we mean programs that grant the same or similar degrees as a proposed new program, or that are required for the proposed new program to function effectively; for instance, a doctoral program in pharmacy would require a successful undergraduate pharmacy program.) In the meantime, resources that might otherwise have been devoted to establishing new programs should be devoted to strengthening those that already exist and to developing the infrastructure needed to support future expansion of training capacity.

Policymakers Should Develop Incentives to Ensure an Appropriate Supply of Qualified Professionals. The Palestinian health system is likely to benefit from the creation of a student loan program for study in accredited health training programs. We understand that many qualified students currently face significant financial barriers to continuing their education, and that Palestinian university students are disproportionately concentrated in the humanities (versus the sciences) in part because the educational fees are lower in those fields. To the extent that training in the health professions represents a good long-term investment—i.e., via more job opportunities and higher earning potential—both the students and Palestinian society would be better off if loans for such study were available.

Loan programs and other forms of support may be particularly valuable in fields where there is an acute shortage of qualified personnel (based on national targets or on operational conditions). The specific fields to be supported should be updated over time to ensure that those with present shortages do not become oversupplied. Under free labor market conditions, labor shortages in particular fields may be self-correcting over time (e.g., because high demand and correspondingly high salaries induce people to enter those fields). However, the large Palestinian government sector may dampen some of these incentives. Also, many Palestinians face liquidity constraints in pursuing education—i.e., they are unable to borrow enough money to pursue relatively expensive training, even if that training would pay off over their professional career.

Palestinian training programs should also be adjusted (for instance, by shifting resources to other areas) in the event of an oversupply of qualified personnel in particular health fields. In addition, the government health system should use flexible compensation and contracting arrangements to reflect the relative demand for personnel with different types of training.

The Public Sector Should Be Able to Attract and Retain an Adequate Number of Appropriately Qualified Staff. Given the current and likely future role of the government as a provider of care in Palestine—and given its administrative, regulatory, and enforcement responsibilities—it is essential that the MOH and other relevant government institutions be able to attract and retain suitably qualified professionals. This may require increasing the salaries of health professionals in the government sector. It may also require changing the civil service law, which is currently relatively weak; ensuring a stable career path for government employees in the health sector; and developing merit-based hiring, retention, and promotion criteria that are consistently applied.

We recognize that any efforts to improve labor conditions in the MOH are likely to have implications for all ministries and public employees. Such changes may be most plausible in the context of broader civil service reforms.

Managers in All Health Sectors Should Receive Appropriate Training, Initially and on an Ongoing Basis. To function effectively, health system managers need to be able to use modern systems for planning, budgeting, procurement, accounting, data collection and analysis, and other key functions. These skills must be continuously maintained and updated. Effective training programs in these areas should be established and strengthened.

Policymakers or Local Institutions Should Develop Cooperative Agreements with Foreign Institutions Regarding Training and Academic Exchange. For a health care system and population the size of Palestine's, any efficient human resource development strategy will include having some people train abroad, rather than attempting to develop all necessary training capacity domestically. In this context, the Palestinian health system is likely to benefit from the development of bilateral agreements with foreign countries and/or institutions to designate training slots for suitably qualified Palestinian students and to enable periodic exchange of faculty.

With respect to training abroad, appropriate institutions should be developed to increase the likelihood that Palestinian students trained abroad will return to work in Palestine, at least for some period of time. There are various international models for this, many of which are already being used by Palestinian organizations that help sponsor foreign training.

Under conditions of peace, training in Israel is likely to be a very cost-effective option for Palestinians, and the exchange may itself contribute to the peace process. In the past, many Palestinian health professionals have received such training; indeed, some Palestinians are currently training in Israeli institutions. Palestinians training in Israel may be able to live at home, or at least to travel home frequently and cheaply. In addition, Palestinians trained in Israel (rather than in other countries) may be more likely to return to Palestine when their training is completed.

Basic Science Education Should Be Improved. Stronger science education at all levels of the Palestinian education system, including primary and secondary schools, would help ensure that future cohorts of Palestinian graduates have the qualifications to pursue health-related training if they choose. Strengthening public education programs is particularly important for poor students, whose opportunities are otherwise especially limited.

Effects of Restricted Domestic Mobility

For human resource development, the problems associated with restricted mobility are analogous to those for the development of health care facilities, services, and programs. Specifically, implementation and enforcement of appropriate licensing and accreditation standards are more difficult; and it is more difficult and costly to develop high-quality education programs if the mobility of students and faculty is restricted.

Effects of Restricted International Access

Licensing and accreditation are generally implemented domestically. However, restricted international access for students and health professionals is likely to hinder strategies for human resource development. It is unlikely that the medical, nursing, public health, and other manpower needs of the new state can all be met domestically at appropriate levels of quality. Meeting these needs is likely to require access to educational institutions in Israel, Jordan, and other countries for Palestinian students and health professionals who seek advanced training (as well as access to Palestine by foreign health professionals who might provide training in Palestinian institutions).

Prior to 2000, for instance, there was regular cooperation between Israeli and Palestinian institutions regarding training of health professionals. Nearly all official cooperation ended following the outbreak of the second intifada, although some activities continue on a personal level. Israeli interview participants told us that their institutions would welcome the resumption and indeed expansion of such cooperation with their Palestinian counterparts, circumstances and resources permitting.

Over time, it is also possible to imagine flows of students into Palestine and flows of Palestinian faculty to foreign institutions. Indeed, the latter, and to some degree the former, already takes place.

Health Care Quality Improvement

Background

Although formal assessment of the quality of health care in Palestine was outside the scope of this analysis, available evidence suggests that patient satisfaction with the Palestinian health care system is low. Patients generally regard health care services in Palestine as inferior, and those who can afford to do so seek care in Jordan, Israel, and elsewhere. Patient satisfaction with private and NGO services is higher than with the government sector, particularly in the last several years when the PA's waiving of government health insurance premiums led to a doubling of enrollment without a corresponding increase in capacity. In our experience, opinions among providers and other health system leaders mirror those of patients. Our interview participants consistently emphasized the need to improve health care quality with respect to primary, secondary, and tertiary care and in all sectors of the health system.

Before and after 1994, many health care quality improvement (QI) projects have been undertaken in Palestine. Some projects were relatively independent, implemented by one organization or facility and often the result of the personal initiative of individual providers. Others were part of systematic QI efforts. These efforts have improved care in specific clinical areas, in specific institutions, and in the health system overall. Indeed, Palestine was one of the first developing areas where modern QI practices were shown to be effective.

Systematic efforts by Palestinian authorities predate the creation of the MOH, beginning with the establishment of the Central Unit for Quality of Health Care within the Palestinian Council of Health in 1994. This unit developed the *Strategic Plan for Quality of Health Care in Palestine* and the *Operational Plan for Quality of Health Care in Palestine*, the overall goals of which were to introduce and institutionalize the use of modern QI methods in the government health sector and in the Palestinian health system generally.

When the Central Unit for Quality of Health Care was discontinued in June 1995, its responsibilities were assumed and expanded by the Quality Improvement Project (QIP) within the MOH. The QIP operated dozens of successful QI projects in several demonstration sites and worked to expand the number of facilities in which it operated. It also provided formal training in QI methods to several hundred health professionals. By the late 1990s, however, the QIP had ceased to function effectively because of lack of institutional support within the MOH and travel restrictions within Palestine. The World Bank's current health-sector development projects in the West Bank and Gaza include QI components.

Although QI projects continue throughout the health system, they are no longer part of a coordinated national process. In general, QI interventions such as clinical practice guidelines or clinical pathways, provider reminder systems, or quality-based financial incentives are not widely used in the Palestinian health system; nor are institutional processes such as continuous QI or total quality management. However, some efforts are currently under way to increase use of evidence-based protocols and guidelines in Palestine, particularly regarding nutrition, diabetes, and maternal and child care. This work has been funded by international donors and is supported by the MOH.

Quality improvement depends on reliable evaluation. A number of organizations within the Palestinian health system have capabilities in program and policy evaluation, including the MOH; Al-Quds and Birzeit Universities and other academic institutions; the Health Development, Information and Policy Institute (HDIP) and other NGOs; and others.[12] However, these existing capacities are weak in a number of important ways. For instance, the number of professional positions available to trained health researchers is relatively limited, so there is insufficient capacity to address all relevant issues. In addition, as is true in many other settings throughout the world, new health-related policies and demonstration programs are often implemented without an explicit evaluation component, and the results of many initiatives are not systematically documented or published.

Recommendation: A National Strategy on Health Care Quality Improvement Should Be Developed and Implemented, with Systematic Evaluation of Quality Improvement Projects and Dissemination of Those That Succeed

Every health care system faces challenges in institutionalizing health care QI processes. However, successful strategies typically include some common features, as described below.

Quality Improvement Efforts Should Be Coordinated. National QI efforts should be coordinated to enhance their efficiency and to facilitate evaluation. In addition, priorities for QI should be consistent with national health planning targets. The national strategic plan for QI should be updated.

Facilities and Programs Should Adopt Systematic, Modern Quality Improvement Processes. In many settings, one key component of QI efforts is adoption of an institutional QI process; e.g., one that uses the principles of total quality management. An institutional process helps create a framework of responsibility within the facility or program for choosing and implementing QI projects and makes such activities part of an organization's core functions.

Quality Improvement Projects Should Be Evidence Based. There is a considerable and expanding literature regarding the efficacy, effectiveness, and cost-effectiveness of

---

[12] HDIP maintains an annotated bibliography of journal articles and other reports on health and health care in Palestine (see Barghouthi, Fragiacomo, and Qutteina, 1999; and Barghouthi, Shubita, and Fragiacomo, 2000).

various QI strategies in health care. Although findings in other geographic areas or practice settings may not always apply to Palestine, this evidence base is likely to provide a valuable frame of reference for local QI efforts, particularly if interventions are carefully adapted to local circumstances.

Quality Improvement Projects Should Be Evaluated, and the Results Should Be Publicized. While some QI projects in Palestine have been formally evaluated, many have not. When programs are evaluated, the results are often not widely disseminated or publicly accessible. Systematic evaluation of QI interventions would help develop an evidence base of best practices in Palestine, which would help guide future health system planning and development. In addition, such evidence would also serve as a useful reference for QI efforts in other developing areas.

Successful Quality Improvement Projects Should Be Supported and Disseminated. In many settings, even successful demonstration projects are not sustained in place after the demonstration period, nor are they widely disseminated. Patients, providers, and other health system stakeholders are likely to benefit if the QI process in Palestine includes explicit strategies for sustaining and spreading QI projects that are found to be cost-beneficial or relatively cost-effective from a societal perspective.

Effects of Restricted Domestic Mobility

Like health system planning and policy development, the ability to carry out and evaluate QI activities would be significantly inhibited under conditions of restricted mobility.

Effects of Restricted International Access

QI activities are generally implemented domestically. However, the development of QI programs would be inhibited if staff responsible for QI activities were unable to travel internationally for training and professional collaboration.

Policies on Prescription Drugs and Medical Devices

Background

Following several years of development, the MOH distributed the first national drug list in 2003. Development of the list was informed by several sources, including the essential drug lists developed by the WHO. The new list is likely to be of considerable value to the Palestinian health system, particularly the government sector, by helping to define its pharmaceutical policy in a public and systematic way. However, the national drug list was distributed without corresponding training for clinicians and pharmacists in how to use the list. In addition, there is currently no systematic process in place for updating the national drug list, although there are several reasons to expect that such updating will be beneficial. Most obviously, new and more effective drugs are frequently introduced. In addition, there is a constant stream of drugs coming off patent. Such drugs should be evaluated for possible inclusion in the formulary. One example is the antidepressant fluoxetine (brand name Prozac), which was on patent and not on the national drug list when the list was originally developed. Although fluoxetine has subsequently come off patent, it remains off the list.

In addition, both the content of the national drug list and the amount of each drug that is purchased and distributed by the MOH were largely based on historical prescribing and consumption patterns in Palestine, with relatively little explicit consideration of scientific evidence on effectiveness, cost-effectiveness, or patterns of microbial resistance. As a result, if past prescribing and consumption patterns were clinically or economically inefficient, the current national drug list—and MOH purchasing policies—are likely to reflect these inefficiencies.

Distribution of pharmaceuticals in the government sector is currently uneven, with excess supply of many drugs in some places (particularly urban centers) and shortages elsewhere. The MOH and the World Bank are currently developing improved pharmaceutical data systems, focusing on inventories and expiration dates. Such systems are likely to be beneficial, particularly if they are integrated with data on geographic patterns of morbidity and patterns of pharmaceutical prescribing and use. However, such data systems do not currently exist.

Although there is a considerable domestic pharmaceutical industry, there has been little coordination between the MOH and pharmaceutical suppliers regarding the domestic supply of drugs on the national drug list—even regarding drugs with a short shelf life and those that are required for treatment of life-threatening conditions. However, a promising recent development is the coordination between the MOH and the United States Agency for International Development (USAID) to develop a program of local procurement of some of the products on the national drug list, with the explicit intent of building strategic reserves for particular medicines.

The uncertain supply of necessary drugs from domestic or foreign sources has created problems for some patients when importation and/or local distribution of pharmaceuticals has been disrupted, as has occasionally occurred since 1994 and particularly since the outbreak of the second intifada.

In 2002, some international donations of pharmaceuticals to the MOH included products that were not on the national drug list. However, the MOH rejected some donations for clinical and policy reasons. International donations also apparently included some products for which there were actually domestic suppliers, effectively undermining Palestinian producers. To our knowledge, the MOH does not have a formal policy for how to handle such donations.

Although responsibility for the Palestinian health system was transferred to the PA in 1994, the PA and MOH do not have complete authority over pharmaceuticals and other medical products. In particular, all such products imported into Palestine must be registered in Israel, using Israeli standards. In our view, this policy results in both potential costs and benefits for Palestine. On the one hand, this policy is likely to raise the cost of pharmaceuticals in Palestine, by limiting potential foreign suppliers to those who have incurred the cost of registering in Israel. On the other hand, it may help ensure the quality of imported drugs. In addition to possible clinical benefits, the local pharmaceutical industry might benefit by closing the Palestinian market to low-quality—and very low priced—competition.

In our interviews, Israeli stakeholders expressed the expectation that Israeli restrictions on Palestinian imports would be eliminated with the establishment of an independent Palestinian state. The MOH currently has a process for licensing pharmaceuticals and other medical products that are locally produced, but it is not as comprehensive as the Israeli process. In any case, the capacities of this process would need to be expanded significantly if responsibility over imported products were also transferred to the PA.

Recommendation: Policymakers Should Implement National Strategies on the Licensing, Supply, and Distribution of Pharmaceuticals and Medical Devices to Ensure a Stable and Adequate Supply of Safe and Cost-Effective Products

Successful strategies in this area are likely to include some common features, as described below.

There Should Be a Systematic Process in Place for Updating the National Drug List. To remain clinically relevant and cost-effective, drug formularies need to be updated periodically to reflect current evidence on clinical efficacy and cost-effectiveness of new and existing drugs, and changes in the supply and cost of particular drugs. Since the national drug list is binding only for the government sector in Palestine, it may be most appropriate for the updating process to be led by the MOH. We recognize that effective implementation of this process is likely to require improved health information systems, particularly regarding microbial resistance (discussed further in the following section).

Products on the National Drug List Should Be Consistently Available Throughout the Government Health System. Consumers and providers are likely to regard the health system as deficient if the drugs to which people are formally entitled as part of their health insurance benefit are not consistently available. A reliable supply will require efficient distribution methods, which in turn will require improved health information systems.

Training for Pharmacists and for Clinicians Regarding Pharmaceuticals Should Be Strengthened. Our interview participants mentioned a number of quality issues, including prescribing without appropriate clinical indications, dispensing without a prescription, dispensing drugs that are past their expiration date, and prescribing and dispensing without adequate instructions for patients. We have already discussed recommendations for improving licensing and continuing education for clinicians, pharmacists, and other health care professionals. Here, we emphasize that initial and continuing training programs regarding pharmaceuticals should focus particularly on the content of the national drug list to ensure that clinicians can prescribe and pharmacists can dispense all these medications appropriately—a level of skill that is not currently universal.

Policymakers Should Review and, If Necessary, Update the National Prescribing Law. The national health plans and many of our interview participants referred to the need for an updated national prescribing law. One specific provision called for in the national health plans is mandatory generic substitution. Although such provisions have been beneficial elsewhere, these and other details should be resolved locally.

It is apparently common practice for pharmacists to dispense prescription medications to patients without a physician's prescription. This is officially prohibited, and this prohibition should be enforced consistently. At the same time, some interview participants suggested that it might be cost-effective for pharmacists to have discretion in recommending specific medications, conditional on receiving diagnosis information and recommending that a patient receive prescriptions from a physician. Such a policy might be beneficial, particularly given the current lack of uniform training and licensing standards among physicians and pharmacists in Palestine.

The National Programs for Licensing Pharmaceuticals, Medical Devices, and Medical Consumables Should Be Strengthened. Every health system should have specific procedures for licensing drugs and other medical products to determine which products may be sold and to ensure that they are safe and effective. As we have described, the Palestinian health system currently relies on Israel to perform much of this function, as part of the agreements in the Oslo process. It may be efficient for the Palestinian health system to incorporate the licensing determinations of Israel or other third parties into its own policies. If so, however, this decision should be made explicitly by local policymakers. Even then, new and expanded responsibilities are likely to fall on the Palestinian health system, and its capabilities in this area will need to be strengthened and expanded.

Effects of Restricted Domestic Mobility

Efficient distribution of pharmaceuticals would be significantly inhibited under conditions of restricted mobility, as has been the case during the second intifada. As discussed above, licensing and education activities would also be inhibited.

Effects of Restricted International Access

Restrictions on international trade would inhibit efficient and clinically appropriate pharmaceutical policies by restricting access to imported pharmaceuticals and to the raw materials needed for domestic pharmaceutical production, and by inhibiting Palestinian exports. Licensing of pharmaceuticals and medical devices would mostly be implemented locally. However, those programs would be inhibited if staff responsible for them were unable to travel internationally for training and professional collaboration.

Health Information Systems

Background

For this analysis, we define "health information systems" relatively widely to include all types of data that are directly relevant to health system planning, operation, and evaluation. These data encompass vital statistics; epidemiological data, including but not limited to nutritional status, vaccine coverage, microbial resistance, behavioral risk factors, incidence of infectious disease, incidence and prevalence of chronic illness, and disease registries; hospital cost and discharge data; data on cost and use of ambulatory care; inventory and consumption data for pharmaceuticals and other medical products; health insurance registry; tracking systems for international referrals; and medical records.

Many of these types of data are currently collected in some fashion in the Palestinian health system. For instance, vital statistics are maintained by the Palestinian Central Bureau of Statistics, which shares these and other data within the government and with outside parties. Many types of epidemiological monitoring have been conducted by the Palestinian Central Bureau of Statistics and the MOH, including population- and clinic-based surveys of nutritional status and vaccine coverage, tracking of infectious disease, and data on the incidence and prevalence of noncommunicable and chronic diseases. Anthropometric status has been included in pediatric medical records in the government health system since the 1980s. Some data are available on use of inpatient and outpatient care, particularly within the government health system.

These data have supported previous national planning efforts, policy development, research, and evaluation. However, the success of future health system development efforts will require significant strengthening of existing systems, the introduction of new data capabilities, and more systematic use of data in informing health system policies and operation.

Perhaps most important, existing data systems have not been developed in an integrated, coordinated fashion. Many types of data that are essential for effective health system planning and operation are not consistently available, including national health accounts that cover all health sectors, comprehensive chronic disease registries, and data on pharmaceutical prescribing and use. Even vital statistics data, which are relatively well developed, have important limitations. For instance, births are recorded by the father's name and are not easily linked to the records of the mother. A related issue is that many types of data are collected in some parts of the health system but not in others and/or are collected in different—and incompatible—formats in different locations. Also, many types of data are recorded on paper rather than electronically.

Some efforts to strengthen particular information systems are currently under way. For instance, Birzeit University and the MOH have developed and are implementing updated pediatric medical records, which improve on previous charts by including screening tools for various developmental conditions. Ongoing, population-based nutritional monitoring is being conducted or supported by various organizations, including Birzeit University, Al-Quds University, Johns Hopkins University, CARE, Maram/USAID, the United Nations Children's Fund, the Palestinian Central Bureau of Statistics, and the Food and Agriculture Organization of the United Nations. The World Bank is currently sponsoring a major project with the MOH to strengthen various health information systems, including national registries for health insurance and international referrals; clinical information (on a pilot basis); and a central repository for health data, which will track data on vaccinations, pharmaceutical inventories, incidence of reportable infectious disease, and—in a subsequent phase—hospital discharge data based on the discharge system of the European Hospital in Gaza.

Since its creation in 2001, the Health Inforum has served as an information clearinghouse for the Palestinian health sector.[13] Among other things, Health Inforum maintains a database of health development projects in Palestine. The materials available through Health Inforum were invaluable for our analyses.

These various efforts should be continued and supported—but these efforts alone are unlikely to meet the information needs of the Palestinian health system.

Recommendation: Palestinian Policymakers Should Develop Comprehensive, Modern, and Integrated Health Information Systems

Successful health information systems are likely to include a number of common features, as described below.

Data Should Be Collected on Incidence and Prevalence of Noncommunicable Diseases and on Behavioral Risk Factors. Currently, available data suggest that incidence and prevalence of noncommunicable diseases are high and rising rapidly, including diabetes, hypertension, heart disease, and cancer. However, data on these conditions are incomplete as a result of considerable undiagnosed morbidity and a lack of comprehensive population-based screening or surveys in these areas. Also, to our knowledge there is currently no national cancer/tumor registry, nor registries for other relevant diseases (including for inheritable genetic conditions, some of which are relatively prevalent in Palestine). Accurate data in these areas are essential for effective health system planning and operation.

The Palestinian health system is also likely to benefit from a surveillance system of behavioral risk factors, including cigarette smoking, diet, and physical activity. There was a consensus among interview participants that health promotion and disease prevention efforts need to be strengthened. For instance, several interview participants mentioned that levels of obesity have apparently been increasing among Palestinians, even during periods of economic crisis; another pointed out that the MOH incurs substantial costs for treating diabetes but currently spends very little on diabetes education. Comprehensive surveillance of behavioral risk factors would help to target and implement interventions.

---

[13] See http://www.healthinforum.net/.

Data Should Be Collected on Nutritional Status, Food Availability, and Food Security. As we have already noted, nutritional status has been and continues to be a key area of concern in Palestine. A number of new data collection initiatives have been implemented in the area of nutritional status, food availability, and food security, including ongoing monitoring reported on a biweekly basis in the Inforum newsletter. Effective monitoring of these issues should be institutionalized. Such data are likely to facilitate health planning and program evaluation.

Health Manpower Registries Should Be Established. Policies to strengthen licensing, certification, and continuing education of health professionals are likely to require national registry systems for all types of health professionals. These systems could track the licensing and certification status of all health professionals eligible to work in Palestine, across all sectors of the health system. They could also track participation in continuing medical education.

National Health Accounts Data Should Be Strengthened. The MOH, the Palestinian Central Bureau of Statistics, Health Inforum, and other sources have worked to create comprehensive and consistent accounts of health system revenue and spending. However, available data need to be improved, particularly regarding international donations (currently, better data are available on pledges than on disbursements) and the private and NGO sectors. The Italian Cooperation is currently sponsoring a project to improve national health accounts.

Hospital Cost and Discharge Data Systems Should Be Strengthened. Stronger national hospital data systems, including systems that capture patterns of cost and use (i.e., discharges), are likely to facilitate improvement of health system management practices. The World Bank and the MOH are planning a development project in this area based on the discharge system of the European Hospital in Gaza. In addition to a hospital discharge system, the Palestinian health system is likely to benefit from a national hospital cost accounting system to be used by both public and private hospitals in Palestine.

Data Should Be Collected on Outpatient Costs and Health Care Use. The MOH and other organizations currently collect and report data on the use of many types of outpatient care. These data are reported, for example, in the annual MOH reports on health in Palestine. However, current data are fairly limited, particularly with respect to costs and services provided in the private and NGO sectors. Enhanced data in these areas are also likely to facilitate health system planning and program evaluation. Comprehensive monitoring of outpatient use and costs may be expensive, and policymakers should balance the benefits of ongoing monitoring against the costs of data collection.

Medical Records and Clinical Screening Systems Should Be Strengthened. As noted above, the MOH and the World Bank are currently piloting an improved clinical information system in a small number of clinics, and the MOH and Birzeit University are developing new pediatric charts. Screening of newborns for phenylketonuria (PKU) and congenital hypothyroidism began during the 1980s, but screening for congenital hip dislocations, heart defects, thalassemia, and other congenital conditions is less common. Similarly, screening of adults for chronic disease risk factors is not currently widespread.

New charts and clinical information systems will require systematically training clinic staff to use the new systems. Improved screening and diagnosis must be accompanied by appropriate follow-up services when problems are detected; these should include treatment referrals, patient education, and social support services.

Pharmacy Data Systems Should Be Strengthened. Improved data on pharmaceutical inventories and use will help to strengthen national pharmaceutical policy. The MOH and the World Bank are currently piloting an information system for primary care clinics that includes a prescription drug module.

Regional and International Systems for Data Exchange Should Be Strengthened. Health in Palestine is closely bound to health in Israel, Egypt, Jordan, and other countries in the region, because many population health issues are common across the region and/or have the potential to cross borders. As a result, these and other relevant countries are likely to benefit from development of ways to rapidly and accurately exchange epidemiological data, particularly regarding infectious disease. Some such mechanisms are currently in place, particularly between the MOH and Israel. However, these mechanisms require strengthening and expansion.

Health Data Should Be Used More Systematically to Inform Policymaking and Management. In general, Palestinian health information systems are likely to be most useful if they are computerized. We recognize that this is likely to involve considerable investment, and that planners must evaluate technologies carefully to maximize the efficiency and sustainability of national data systems.

Effects of Restricted Domestic Mobility

Restricted mobility would inhibit or prevent the collection of most types of data described in this subsection.

Effects of Restricted International Access

Regional and international systems of data exchange will be more difficult to implement effectively if Palestinian professionals have limited access to foreign countries, particularly Israel or Jordan. Other health information systems are mostly implemented domestically.

Research

Background

Several universities and NGOs in Palestine currently conduct public health and health services research. However, these existing capacities are weak for the same reasons that evaluation capacity is weak. (Evaluation capacity was discussed above, in "Health Care Quality Improvement.") Moreover, there are currently few established clinical or basic science research programs in Palestine. The lack of such programs is likely to limit medical education and efforts to improve clinical care, particularly secondary and tertiary care.

Recommendation: Palestinian Policymakers Should Develop National Strategies Regarding Public Health, Health Services, Clinical, and Basic Science Research

Such strategies are important complements to the national health plans and the *National Plan for Human Resource Development and Education in Health*. Indeed, there is explicit overlap with components of these plans.

We recognize that the Palestinian health system faces significant resource constraints and that efforts to develop research capacity must be realistic and appropriate in this context. However, systematic expansion of research capacity is likely to have a number of benefits for the Palestinian health system. For instance, in addition to producing output that is scientifically valuable *per se,* clinical research programs are likely to contribute to the training of future clinicians and health system leaders. They may help foster international respect for Palestinian institutions, as the Israeli Weizman Institute of Science illustrates with respect to Israeli institutions. Research programs may also help generate revenue.[14] In addition to the Weizman Institute, other local models might include the Lebanese Council for Scientific Research and the Jordanian Higher Council of Science and Technology.

Strategies to develop health research capacity in Palestine will require cooperation among government, academic institutions, NGOs, and international donors. Cooperation regarding research and training with centers of excellence in Israel and other neighboring countries is also likely to be very beneficial.

Many Palestinians with relevant skills currently live abroad, and efforts should be made to recruit members of the Palestinian Diaspora to visit or work at Palestinian research institutions. Also, Palestinian research programs are likely to benefit considerably from international partnerships, for instance with Israeli and Jordanian organizations; among other benefits, such partnership may help attract external research funding.

Effects of Restricted Domestic Mobility

The effect of restricted mobility on research programs will vary by the type of research. In particular, research involving population-based data collection will be inhibited. Basic science and some clinical research depends less on population access and would correspondingly be less affected (although, of course, the researchers themselves need to be able to reach their jobs). As described above, restricted mobility will inhibit the economic viability of a Palestinian state and correspondingly reduce the resources available for research.

---

[14] Interview participants particularly mentioned inheritable genetic disorders as an area where there might be considerable demand—and external financing—for scientific collaboration with international institutions, because of the relatively high prevalence of some such conditions among Palestinians.

Effects of Restricted International Access

As with other areas of human resource development, successful development of Palestinian research capability will require that Palestinian students and faculty have access to foreign institutions and that Palestinian institutions be able to recruit foreign faculty (and, to a lesser degree, students).

Programs for Rapid Improvement

Background

As we noted at the beginning of this book, our principal analytic focus is on the institutions that would be needed for the successful operation of the Palestinian health system over the first decade of a future independent Palestinian state. Given this mid- to long-term policy perspective, we have so far included relatively little discussion of the type and quality of health services being provided in Palestine. We believe that strengthening the "macro-level" institutions on which we have focused will ultimately increase the efficiency and effectiveness of health care and improve health status throughout Palestine.

In this section, however, we diverge from our general approach and consider several specific programs that would directly and rapidly improve the health and health care of Palestinians. There are several reasons for this shift in focus. Rapid improvements are, of course, worthwhile in their own right. In addition, improving health conditions in the short run may also help to achieve longer-run development goals.

At a macro level, social conditions in Palestine since 1994—including health—have not improved as much as many people had hoped or expected. Many factors have contributed to this lack of improvement, including political and armed conflict, but also ineffective governance and weak policy development and implementation. The lack of improvement has certainly undermined support for the PA and its institutions and for the peace process overall. Indeed, many interview participants and other observers suggested that the slow improvement in quality of life for many Palestinians contributed directly to the outbreak of the second intifada.

At a more micro level, a dual strategy of pairing short- and longer-term development efforts may contribute to staff and organizational morale. Interview participants noted that boosting morale is particularly important for organizations that place heavy emphasis on humanitarian assistance in response to current conditions. Indeed, we encountered many organizations that were pursuing projects with various planning horizons, from immediate humanitarian aid to multiyear efforts to develop human and physical infrastructure. Overall, we were consistently impressed by the scope of both short- and long-term development projects that we observed.

In sum, whatever the strengths of the Palestinian health system, there are clearly acute areas of need, and all stakeholders are likely to benefit by addressing them effectively and rapidly. In this context, we make the following recommendations.

Recommendation: The MOH Should Implement Comprehensive Programs to Improve Nutritional Status, Including Food Fortification, Micronutrient Supplementation for High-Risk Groups, and Promotion of Healthy Dietary Practices

Available evidence suggests an urgent need to improve nutritional status in Palestine. Studies have shown persistently high levels of anemia at all ages, based on blood testing and dietary intake studies; malnutrition, particularly among children via anthropometric monitoring; vitamin A deficiency, based on dietary intake studies (a blood study of vitamin A is currently pending); and other nutritional problems. Moreover, there is some evidence that the rates of micronutrient deficiency and malnutrition have increased since the outbreak of the second intifada. Poor nutritional status is a well-recognized cause of short- and long-term health problems across the lifespan, including complications of pregnancy, birth defects, heart disease, cancer, osteoporosis, and other conditions. It also impairs children's psychomotor development and later educational performance, including delay in school enrollment, increased absenteeism, impaired concentration, and increased susceptibility to infectious disease—issues that are less commonly emphasized in the development of nutrition policies.

Although a number of efforts to strengthen nutritional status—and the nutrition policies of the MOH—are currently under way, these efforts needed to be consolidated, expanded, and institutionalized. Such efforts will require cooperation among the MOH, UNRWA, and other stakeholders to develop and implement coordinated, comprehensive national programs to improve nutritional status in Palestine, particularly among children and women of childbearing age. Based on scientific evidence, these programs should include fortification of common foodstuffs with vitamins A and D, iron, and folic acid (folate); and provision of vitamin and mineral supplements to children at least through age two and to childbearing women before, during, and after pregnancy. The government health system provided such supplements to infants in the past, but this practice was discontinued in the mid-1990s. The need for supplements prior to pregnancy would be reduced by an effective national fortification program that includes folate.

Recommendation: The National Immunization Program Should Be Updated, and the Costs of Purchasing and Distributing Vaccines Should Be Explicitly Covered by the Government Budget

Immunization programs have been one of the great strengths of the Palestinian health system since the 1970s, with high coverage of a progressive program of vaccines. However, the Palestinian vaccination schedule needs to be updated somewhat, particularly to reflect the availability of new vaccines such as hepatitis A, haemophilus influenza B, and varicella. Each of these is now included in the Israeli vaccination program.

For several years following 1994, the MOH budget explicitly provided for purchase and distribution of all vaccines covered by the national immunization program. However, this practice was discontinued in response to budget pressures, and the immunization program has subsequently relied on international donations of vaccines.

In our view, the latter practice is unlikely to guarantee the continuous availability of high-quality vaccines to the Palestinian health system, and the former policy should be reinstated.

Recommendation: The MOH and Other Stakeholders Should Expand the Scope of Available Primary Care Services and Expand Access to Comprehensive Primary Care

As we have described, primary care is the current and intended future cornerstone of the Palestinian health care system. However, certain aspects of primary care—as it is commonly defined—require considerable strengthening. These include health promotion and disease prevention, which also need to be strengthened in schools and elsewhere in society; screening and diagnosis, particularly of child developmental disorders and adult chronic and noncommunicable diseases; reproductive health services, including family planning; and psychosocial support and mental health care, for which there are both considerable societal need and a particular shortage of appropriately trained providers. Efforts to strengthen these areas will require cooperation across stakeholders, including the MOH, UNRWA, relevant NGOs, and international donors.

The relative importance of the primary health care delivery system has increased since the outbreak of the second intifada, because primary care clinics are widely distributed and thus relatively accessible during periods of restricted mobility. Geographic closures have also strengthened the role of nurses and other nonphysician professionals, because these staff tend to live closer to the primary care clinics and have been more consistently available to patients than physicians during periods of closure. Some interview participants regarded the resulting change in practice patterns as beneficial for patients, even if it arose for negative reasons. However, interview participants expressed concern that, when closures lift and economic conditions improve, the MOH and other providers are likely to shift resources away from primary care and toward secondary and tertiary care. In our view, such a shift would be both clinically and economically undesirable for the Palestinian health system.

In the short run, efforts to strengthen health promotion and disease prevention could include additional training and empowerment of health educators, social workers, skilled lay people such as village health workers, community groups, and others. However, the number of such people is currently limited and should be increased over time. Key substantive issues to be addressed include public health issues such as sanitation and water quality; traffic, home, and workplace safety; diet and nutrition; physical activity; cigarette smoking; domestic violence; and clinical issues such as developmental disorders, psychosocial problems, and chronic illness.

There is also a need to strengthen treatment programs—sometimes referred to as "tertiary prevention"—for chronic diseases, particularly diabetes, heart disease, and hypertension. As we understand it, these areas have received relatively little emphasis from NGOs and international donors. However, they represent a considerable and increasing fraction of the overall burden of disease among Palestinians. Moreover, there is increasing scientific evidence that many of these conditions can be effectively—and cost-effectively—managed in primary care.[15]

Recommendation: The MOH and Other Stakeholders Should Develop Comprehensive Strategies for Addressing Psychosocial Needs, Particularly Those Relating to the Exposure of Children to Violence

There is an urgent need to strengthen psychosocial support to help mitigate the consequences of the physical, economic, social, and political stressors that have been prevalent in Palestine. Perhaps most notably, there has been considerable exposure to violence from armed conflict, particularly since the start of the second intifada. Yet there is very limited capacity in the health system—and in the education system and other parts of society—to address the developmental and other consequences of these stressors.

One important step is to strengthen psychosocial support and mental health care in primary care, as noted above. However, successful efforts to address psychosocial needs should extend beyond the health care delivery system. In particular, psychological and developmental problems are stigmatized in Palestine, as elsewhere. Patients and family members may not recognize such problems or view them as treatable, and they may be reluctant to seek care in any case. Providers may not diagnose problems correctly, particularly if patients present with somatic complaints; and they may not recommend effective treatment. For these and other reasons, successful strategies are likely to require community-wide collaboration, involving various parts of the health system, the school system, religious institutions, community groups, and other stakeholders. They should include screening, outreach, and other proactive strategies. Proactive strategies are generally valuable for addressing psychosocial problems and particularly for treating psychological trauma; indeed, relatively few trauma victims receive effective care in the absence of outreach programs.

Several relevant programs already exist, including clinic- and school-based programs to address issues among children. These efforts should be continued, but most such programs that we know of are small (one notable exception is the Classroom-Based Intervention program, sponsored by USAID). More generally, we note that the WHO began a new program in 2003 focusing on improving mental health in Palestine. Addressing unmet psychosocial needs will require major increases in qualified personnel, including psychiatrists, psychologists, social workers, school counselors, and qualified lay workers. It will also require the development, dissemination, and support of effective intervention strategies for addressing particular problems, such as psychological trauma among children.

---

[15] These issues are also discussed above, in the context of health care finance and quality improvement.

Effects of Restricted Domestic Mobility

Restricted mobility would inhibit successful achievement of all the recommendations in this section. Both nutrition and immunization initiatives require transport of supplies and personnel, which will be more difficult under restricted mobility. Similarly, training—whether of health professionals or of consumers—will be more difficult to implement successfully.

As we have described, the role of primary care increases under conditions of restricted mobility, because primary care facilities are more widely accessible. Under such circumstances, however, primary care clinics will necessarily emphasize curative care, and there is likely to be little opportunity to expand the scope of care in the areas described above. Similarly, it will be more difficult to expand systems of psychosocial care under conditions of restricted mobility, because training, planning, and implementation will be inhibited. Moreover, as discussed above, restricted mobility is likely to reduce the economic viability of the state, and with it the resources available for expanding health system capacity.

Effects of Restricted International Access

All the services discussed in this section would mainly be provided domestically. However, as with other areas of health system development, the expanded capabilities recommended here will be easier to achieve if Palestinian health professionals have access to technical assistance from abroad and to training in foreign institutions.

CHAPTER SEVEN

Priorities and Timing

As we have described, we believe that the specific priorities for health system development should be determined locally. To this end, we have focused on describing institutions, policies, and programs that are essential for local stakeholders to be able to undertake such priority setting effectively.

In this context, we believe that Palestinian health system development efforts should begin with our first area of emphasis: establishing a planning and coordination authority with adequate power to develop and implement national policy for the Palestinian health system. Indeed, nearly all our interview participants expressed the view that this should occur immediately, not just when an independent Palestinian state is established.

The planning and coordination body would be responsible for reforming policies regarding health insurance and health care finance. It would also oversee the establishment and strengthening of the key institutions described in most of our other recommendations; i.e., licensing and certification of health professionals; licensing and accreditation of facilities, programs, and educational institutions; implementation of national quality improvement strategies; oversight of pharmaceuticals; and collection of national health data.

While we recognize that resources will be scarce, we believe that these institutions are all essential for the successful development of the Palestinian health system. However, the level of available resources will certainly affect the policies and priorities that these institutions pursue. For this reason, among others, we recommend that major new infrastructure projects be deferred until the relevant institutions are in place to ensure that projects are consistent with national priorities and can be implemented effectively.

With respect to research, we believe that efforts to establish research capabilities could begin at any time, and that these capabilities should grow slowly but steadily. Finally, the "rapid improvement" recommendations made in the last section of Chapter Six should be implemented as soon as possible because they have the potential to produce tangible improvements in quality of life for many Palestinians.

CHAPTER EIGHT

Cost

One objective of RAND's project is to estimate the costs involved in strengthening the institutions of a future independent Palestinian state. A general estimate is provided below. However, a detailed estimate of the costs associated with implementing the recommendations made in this book is outside the scope of our analysis. Such an estimate will depend on the specific policy choices that local stakeholders make to address each recommendation, which of course are currently unknown, and on details of the current system that were unavailable for this analysis. For instance, the cost of licensing and accrediting health care facilities or educational programs will depend on the licensing and accreditation standards that are ultimately selected for Palestine and on the extent to which current facilities and programs fall short of those standards. Although we could estimate the cost of the licensing and accreditation process *per se*, using this cost alone is likely to be misleading. The costs of upgrading to meet new standards are likely to dwarf the costs of reviewing programs and of approving or denying their license/accreditation.

In this chapter, we therefore consider health system development costs from a macro perspective. Our policy recommendations in this book focus primarily on incremental reforms to the Palestinian health system, rather than on radical restructuring. As a frame of reference for considering the scale of future investments in the Palestinian health system, we therefore consider two kinds of information: recent levels of per-capita health system spending in Palestine and the level of health system development efforts since 1994.

In 1998, prior to the second intifada, total annual Palestinian health spending was estimated at $100–$111 per capita. Since the start of the second intifada, economic conditions have declined dramatically. Health sector spending has correspondingly declined, although exact data on current per-capita health sector spending are not available. For present purposes we assume a current level of spending of $67 per person per year, 60 percent of the pre-intifada level.[1]

---

[1] Based on data from PA MOH, 2003a, Palestinian gross national income (approximately equivalent to GNP) was $1,070 per capita in 2002, 60 percent of the level reported for 2000. To our knowledge, the MOH has not reported national health expenditures for 2001 or 2002; for present purposes, we assume that per-capita health spending has fallen in proportion to national income.

According to World Bank data for 1997–2000, annual per-capita spending of $111 is very close to the average expenditure of $116 observed among "middle income" countries, as defined by the World Bank; higher than the level observed among "lower middle income" countries ($72); and about one-third the level observed among "upper middle income" countries ($309). Palestinian gross national product per capita ($1,771 in 2000) compares similarly with that of "middle income" countries ($1,860), while "lower middle income" ($1,230) and "upper middle income" ($4,550) countries vary accordingly. In terms of other countries in the region, per-capita health spending of $111 is higher than that reported for Syria ($30) and Egypt ($51), but it is lower than per-capita spending in Jordan ($137), Saudi Arabia ($448), Lebanon ($499), and Israel ($2,021).

The 1998 level of per-capita spending corresponded to total annual health sector expenditures of $320 million to $344 million (given a population of approximately 3.1 million). Of these expenditures, approximately $40 million per year came in the form of international aid. International donations to the Palestinian health system totaled approximately $227 million between 1994 and 2000, an average of $38 million per year. For comparison, disbursement of international donations across all sectors in Palestine was $3.1 billion over the same period, an average of $512 million per year. Thus, slightly over 7 percent of total international donations were directed to the health system. Since the start of the second intifada, considerable international contributions to the health sector have continued, but their focus has shifted a great deal toward humanitarian relief. Detailed information on the distribution of health sector expenditures between operating expenses and capital investment is unavailable; based on available data, however, we estimate that capital investment was on the order of $40 million to $50 million per year.

In this context, we estimate that a constructive level of external support for the Palestinian health system over the first decade of an independent state would be $130 million to $165 million per year, in year 2003 U.S. dollars. Over the ten-year period 2005–2014, this level of external support would total $1.3 billion to $1.65 billion.

This estimate is based on the assumption that the Palestinian health system will require a relatively large amount of resources in the first year or two of an independent state to restore per-capita spending to pre-intifada levels and beyond. At a conceptual level, at least, we regard the pre-intifada level of spending as a sustainable baseline under conditions of peace.

In terms of health sector improvement, we estimate that such contributions would support increasing annual per-capita health sector spending from the estimated current level of $67 to between $122 and $197 per person per year. This estimated effect on per-capita spending assumes that increases in external contributions following the establishment of an independent Palestinian state would be accompanied by increases in other health sector funding (i.e., taxes, insurance premiums, co-payments, and private investments/donations). The higher per-capita spending estimate ($197) assumes that these other funding sources would grow enough to keep the fraction of total health sector spending contributed by external funding at the 1998 level (13.2 percent, or approximately $45 million in external funding out of total health sector spending of $340 million). The lower per-capita spending estimate ($122) assumes that domestic funding sources would rise disproportionately more slowly than external sources, and that the latter would make up three times that proportion of new health sector spending.

Estimated effects on per-capita spending assume an initial population of 3.5 million people (i.e., approximately the current level), and a population growth rate of 4 percent per year (consistent with recent trends). If the annual rate of population growth were 3 percent, this level of external support would increase per-capita spending to between $130 and $217 per person per year (maintaining all other assumptions). Our estimates do not account for "health care inflation"—i.e., the tendency (particularly in developed countries) for health care costs to increase, principally because of the introduction of new products and procedures.

Our estimates are informed by, and broadly consistent with, previously published estimates of the resources needed for health sector development. In particular, in the Palestinian development plan, 1999, the PA estimated that donations of about $60 million per year would be needed for development of the government health sector during 1999–2003. This is about half again as much per year as the average annual level of donations during 1994–2000, and more than twice the annual level of donations that went to the government sector during that period (the rest went to NGOs and UNRWA). A separate calculation for the health system overall, presented in Barnea and Husseini (2002), estimated that the shortfall between health system revenues and the expenditures needed to maintain the system at 1998 levels was between $50 million and $100 million per year for 2001–2004. The amount increases over time because of population growth.[2]

If spent effectively, external support of $130 million to $165 million per year should yield tangible improvements in the Palestinian health system. In terms of per-capita spending, the Palestinian health system would remain below those of some of its more economically advanced neighbors, such as Lebanon, Saudi Arabia, and Israel. Further donations might raise the standards of the health system further. At the same time, this level of external support is three to four times the average annual level of international donations from 1994 to 2000. We believe that the Palestinian health system would have difficulty successfully absorbing international donations of much more than this, and that higher donations would risk waste and disruption (e.g., because of capacity constraints in human and physical capital). Over time, as the Pal-

---

[2] These estimates were prepared prior to the second intifada. Since then, tax revenues, health insurance premiums, and household incomes (which support patients' out-of-pocket spending) all decreased substantially. Deficit estimates under these circumstances would have been correspondingly higher.

estinian health system—and the Palestinian economy—becomes more advanced, its ability to absorb and use outside investments efficiently will increase.

We note that, if responsibility for the health system of East Jerusalem were transferred to a future Palestinian state, additional resources would be needed to maintain current patterns of care and reimbursement in East Jerusalem. This issue requires separate analysis that is outside the scope of this book. Similarly, water and sanitation infrastructure is excluded from this analysis.

Finally, we have based these analyses on data regarding total and per-capita health system spending for Palestine and other areas. We could not determine definitively whether these data capture spending in all areas addressed in this book. If particular areas, such as educational programs for health professionals or research, are generally excluded from these data, our estimates of constructive levels of external support for the Palestinian health system would correspondingly need to be revised.

CHAPTER NINE

Discussion

In this book, we have described a variety of options for strengthening particular aspects of the Palestinian health system, with the goal of improving health and health care for the Palestinian people in the context of an independent Palestinian state. Our recommendations (summarized in Table 6.1) were developed based on considerable input from Palestinian, Israeli, and international professionals who are currently involved in the Palestinian health system or were involved in the past.

Considerable effort will be required to implement the recommendations we have described. In our view, however, such developments are well within the reach of the Palestinian health system, assuming that the larger political and security environment is favorable and that resources are available. Whenever interview participants described a particular policy or project that they felt was important for the Palestinian health system, we asked what they thought would be required to achieve it. Interview participants consistently expressed the view that the necessary human resources existed in Palestine (and among Palestinians living abroad) or could be created relatively quickly—as long as there was a political will among Palestinians to do so, adequate financial resources were available, and the geographic closures ended. We could not verify this view independently. However, the many positive aspects of health and health care in Palestine certainly provide evidence of the considerable skill and motivation of Palestinian health professionals and other stakeholders.

Role of International Donors

International donors have made considerable contributions to the development of the Palestinian health system. In order for the development efforts we have described to be feasible, international donors will need to remain involved for the foreseeable future. Indeed, they will probably need to increase their levels of investment in the health system.

At the same time, we believe that the returns on this investment, in terms of health status and satisfaction with the health system, are likely to be increased if the actions of the donor community are guided by effective local institutions. To this end, care should be taken to use international support to enhance but not replace the responsibility of the MOH and other national institutions for the Palestinian health system. In particular, international support for the Palestinian health system should be closely related to the priorities and targets described in this book, to minimize conflict between the national agenda—which is ultimately a government responsibility—and the agendas of particular donors or NGOs. In turn, international donors could use progress toward reforms described in this book as benchmarks to gauge whether the MOH and other key institutions are performing effectively.

Limitations of Our Analysis

We recognize that this analysis has a number of important limitations. We sought input from a relatively large number of people involved in or knowledgeable about the Palestinian health system, including people from each sector of the health system, academia, international donor organizations, and relevant Israeli institutions. However, our list of interview participants was neither representative nor exhaustive. For instance, because of travel and time restrictions, we had limited in-person contact with MOH personnel; much interaction took place by telephone. We did not interview health care providers employed in the government health sector or representatives of consumer groups or community organizations. We did not speak with any representatives of Islamic organizations, although Islamic NGOs do play an important role in delivering health care and other social services in Palestine.

The input we received was generally consistent across interview participants. However, it is certainly possible that the stakeholders we did not meet would have provided different information. In addition, we did not attempt to validate the accuracy of the information provided by interview participants, beyond comparing comments to information from other interviews, to published reports, and to our own prior experience. Moreover, many of the reports we reviewed were written by one or more of our interview participants, so that these different sources of information were not entirely independent.

In Closing

Our analysis is intended to inform the health system development efforts of a future independent Palestinian state. Outside analyses—including those conducted by international donors and by research organizations such as RAND—can be valuable. However, we believe that successful health system development in Palestine requires that local stakeholders be committed to and in control of both the overall development process and its substantive details.

Selected Objectives from Prior Palestinian Health Plans

Table A.1 presents objectives from several different substantive areas to illustrate the types of goals included in previous national health plans. Goals are for the period 1999–2003.

Table A.2 presents strategies in the previous national health plan's three main substantive areas. Goals are for the period 2001–2006.

Table A.1
Selected Objectives from the 1999 *National Strategic Health Plan*

Area	Recommendation
Health planning and projects management	Develop national sustainable capacity in health planning, policy development, and project management
	Create an information base for health planning and projects management
	Develop measurable indicators to monitor and evaluate planned activities and programs
	Validate community participation, involvement, and ownership initiated during the process of developing the five-year health plan in all Palestinian districts
	Assist in the development of an organized national system for coordination of health developmental activities
	Develop rational master plans for different categories of hospitals and primary health care facilities
	Develop a national accreditation system for planning health sector facilities
Health management information systems	Develop nationwide computerized communication links facilitating the operation of an effective health management information system to be connected to the national information system that links all Palestinian ministries
	Serve the Palestinian community by a system that collects, tabulates, stores, and makes available information on demography, health status, and health resources for policymakers in the health area
	Develop a well-functioning computerized medical information system at district, regional, and central levels by establishing medical information systems in the West Bank and strengthening the existing one in Gaza
	Develop and implement an extensive training program for selected health personnel representing major health care professions from different settings, including the MOH, hospitals, and primary health care
Health promotion and education: chronic heart disease/stroke	Reduce by 40 percent the level of ill health and death caused by heart disease and stroke
	Reduce by 60 percent the risks associated with heart disease by modifying specific human behaviors
Health promotion and education: maternal and child health	Reduce infant mortality from 24.2 in 1997 to 15 deaths per 1,000 live births
	Reduce maternal mortality and morbidity by 50 percent
	Reduce prenatal and neonatal deaths by 50 percent
	Increase by 50 percent the utilization rate of maternal and child health services, especially postnatal care, throughout Palestine
	Increase vaccination coverage to 100 percent, especially tetanus toxoid for teenagers

SOURCE: PA MOH, 1999.

Table A.2
Selected Objectives from the 2001 *National Plan for Human Resource Development and Education in Health*

Area	Recommendation
Planning for health care human resources in Palestine	Conduct national health planning for the various health professions
	Prepare and/or update databases on health care human resources in Palestine
	Develop national and institutional capacities in health planning and development
	Develop and utilize scientific research in health planning and human resource development and promote decision-linked research in human resource development
	Explore fields of cooperation in planning and human resource development at the national, regional, and international levels
	Improve the image of some health-related professions (e.g., nursing, midwifery, and occupational therapy)
Education and training of human resources	Develop and implement an accreditation system for formal education/training programs of health human resources
	Conduct continuing education activities involving the different health professions' categories based on continuing education priority needs as indicated in Welfare Association, PA, and Ministry of Higher Education, 2001a–f
	Provide scholarships within the next five years for priority specialty qualifications in selected health professions
	Strengthen available academic programs and start new programs according to priorities indicated in Welfare Association, PA, and Ministry of Higher Education, 2001a–f
	Start, upgrade, and develop databases on formal degree-granting educational programs in health
	Utilize technology and varied nontraditional teaching-learning methodologies in educational programs
	Develop continuing education potential
	Strengthen clinical/practical training to support educational programs in health
	Develop a remedial training program for physicians and programs for other health care professionals who need such training
Management of health care human resources	Develop conducive managerial practices in health care human resource development
	Ensure availability of necessary protocols/guidelines/rules and regulations related to human resource development
	Strengthen professional unions/associations and health-related councils to promote human care resource development
	Promote an organizational climate that enhances continuing education and human resource development

SOURCE: Welfare Association, PA, and Ministry of Higher Education, 2001a–f.

Methods

The analyses underlying this book were mainly conducted between December 2002 and July 2003.

First, we reviewed previously published academic research and policy analyses regarding health and health care in Palestine to understand the history of the Palestinian health system and the current status of health and health care in Palestine.[1] These materials were available in the form of books, journal articles, reports by government organizations (i.e., the Palestinian and Israeli Ministries of Health), reports by international organizations (e.g., the World Bank, various United Nations agencies, the World Health Organization), reports by Palestinian and international nongovernmental organizations, scientific publications, conference proceedings, working papers, and other formats. We reviewed all such information that we could obtain, with the goal of identifying priorities for health system development in Palestine over the next decade.

Second, we identified and contacted local stakeholders in Palestine and Israel whose input we wanted regarding this analysis, based on their expertise in the organization, operation, and financing of the Palestinian health system. We interviewed each of these experts several times by telephone. Given our project mandate, each person was asked to identify priorities for health system development in Palestine over the next decade. We discussed these issues iteratively with each expert, along with issues we identified from our literature review. We did not use an interview guide for these discussions.

In addition, we asked each expert to recommend additional people whom we could ask for information regarding the Palestinian health system and our analysis. We specifically asked to be referred to people in all sectors of the Palestinian health system; relevant Palestinian and Israeli academics; and people from relevant international organizations, particularly key donors to the Palestinian health system.[2] We tried to contact

---

[1] We include a partial listing in the bibliography. See also the HDIP annotated bibliography of journal articles and other reports on health and health care in Palestine (Barghouthi, Fragiacomo, and Qutteina, 1999; and Barghouthi, Shubita, and Fragiacomo, 2000).

[2] The European Union is sponsoring a comprehensive health sector review on behalf of the PA MOH that overlaps in time and subject with RAND's analysis. We discuss this in additional detail in Appendix D.

everyone to whom we were referred. In addition, we decided that it was important to interview certain categories of stakeholders to whom we had not already been referred. They fell into two broad categories: international organizations, particularly donors, and Palestinian women active in health care delivery and health policy. We identified people in these categories through a combination of referral and independent research.

In March and April, 2003, we contacted the people to whom we had been referred by fax, mail, email, and/or telephone. We provided materials describing this project, including its background and aims, along with a preliminary list of health system development priorities and a general set of questions we wanted to discuss with them (a sample letter of introduction is included as Appendix C of this book). We asked people to meet with us during a visit to Palestine and Israel in May 2003. We scheduled meetings with everybody who said they would be available. No person whom we approached about this project explicitly refused to meet with us, although some people were unavailable for various reasons.

In March 2003, we also held a two-day meeting at RAND's office in Washington, D.C. During that meeting, we discussed the information in the written materials we had reviewed, and we discussed our analysis plans and the strategy for our upcoming trip with several Palestinian and Israeli experts.

In May 2003, Drs. Schoenbaum and Deckelbaum traveled to Palestine and Israel for two weeks.[3] Together with Timea Spitka, we met with the majority of the local stakeholders to whom we had been referred. Nearly all meetings took place face-to-face in Jerusalem or Ramallah. Because Gaza was closed to foreigners during the entire period of this visit, meetings with the Palestinian Ministry of Health in Gaza, and with other relevant stakeholders of that area, had to be postponed or canceled. Where possible, these interviews were conducted by telephone instead, and we were subsequently able to meet with one Gaza contact in Washington, D.C.

In each interview, the questions listed in the letter of introduction served as a general interview guide (see Appendix C). Interview questions were open-ended, so as not to constrain the scope of the information that people provided. Interview participants were asked to base their responses on their own expertise and experience.

Interview participants were asked to allow themselves to be identified in this book. However, to help ensure that people felt free to express their views fully, interview participants were assured that no comments would be quoted directly, or attributed to them in an identifiable way. We took written notes during all meetings, which we subsequently transcribed. Only we and Timea Spitka had access to the meeting notes. The list of interview participants is included at the end of this appendix.

All interview participants received a draft version of this book and were invited to submit comments prior to publication. They were told that we would seriously con-

---

[3] Adel Afifi was also scheduled to participate in this trip, but he was unable to do so because of a family emergency.

sider all comments but not necessarily implement them in the final book. This book was also reviewed in accordance with RAND's usual quality assurance procedures.

The following people were interviewed for this book:

Hani Abdeen, Al-Quds University
Ziad Abdeen, Al-Quds University
Haidar Abdel-Shafi, Palestine Red Crescent Society
Yehia Abed, Maram
Mahmoud Abu-Hadid, Al-Quds University
Fathi Abumoghli, Palestine Ministry of Health (in association with the World Bank)
Zeid M. Abu Shawish, Palestine Ministry of Health
Hikmat Ajjuri, Palestinian Council of Health
Mamdouh M. Aker
Younis Al-Khatib, Palestine Red Crescent Society
Mirca Barbolini, European Union
Mustafa Barghouthi, Union of Palestinian Medical Relief Committees
Tamara Barnea, JDC-Brookdale Institute
Sherry F. Carlin, United States Agency for International Development
Ellan Coates, Maram
Khuloud Dajani, Al-Quds University
Nahil Dajani, Dajani Maternity Hospital
Rajai Dajani, Dajani Maternity Hospital
Anwar Dudin, Al-Quds University
Rita Giacaman, Birzeit University
P. Gregg Greenough, Johns Hopkins University
Arafat S. Hidmi, Makassed Charitable Society
Rafaella Iodice, European Union
Emil Jarjoui, Palestine Liberation Organization
Anne Johansen, World Bank
Salam Kanaan, World Bank
Umaya Khamash, Maram
Rana Khatib, Birzeit University
Bassim Khoury, Pharmacare PLC
Hanan Halabi, Birzeit University
Samia Haleleh, Birzeit University
Abdullatif S. Husseini, Birzeit University
Rafiq Husseini, Welfare Association
Ajay Mahal, Harvard University
Faris Massoud
Rashad Massoud, University Research Co. LLC
Shlomo Mor-Yosef, Hadassah Medical Organization
Salva Najab, Maram

Joumana Odeh, Happy Child Center
As'ad Ramlawi, Palestine Ministry of Health
Ann Roberts, Maram
Yitzhak Sever, Israel Ministry of Health
Mohammad Shahin, Al-Quds Medical School
Varsen Aghabekian Shahin, Al-Quds University
Toufik Shakhshir
Munther Al Sharif, Palestine Ministry of Health
Hossam K. Sharkawi, Palestine Red Crescent Society
Raghda Shawa
Husam E. Siam, UNRWA
Ricardo Solé Arqués, World Health Organization
Suzy Srouji, United States Agency for International Development
Theodore Tulchinsky, Hebrew University School of Public Health
Henrik Wahlberg, World Health Organization
Laura Wick, Birzeit University

Letter of Introduction Regarding RAND's Health System Analysis

<date>

Dear Sir or Madam:

We are writing to you on behalf of RAND, an independent, non-partisan research organization based in California. With the support of private donors, RAND is analyzing important parameters for the success of a future independent Palestinian state. RAND will distribute the findings from this research to key policy-makers in the United States, Palestine and Israel.

As part of this larger project, our working group is leading an analysis of the Palestinian health system. Our goals are: 1) to understand the strengths and gaps of the current system, with respect to organization, human and physical infrastructure, and financing; 2) to identify major priorities for future development and investment, over approximately the next ten years; and 3) to estimate the financial cost of reaching various development goals.

We are currently planning to visit the region in May to meet with key Palestinian, Israeli and international stakeholders. We would like to speak or meet with you as part of our work. In the meantime, we would like to provide more information about our project and RAND.

About RAND and RAND Health

RAND is an independent, non-profit research organization, with headquarters in Santa Monica, California, and other main offices in Washington, Pittsburgh, and Leiden (the Netherlands). RAND was established in 1948. RAND's mission is to improve policy and decision-making through research and analysis. RAND has a staff of more than 1600. 85% of the research staff hold advanced degrees, with more than 65% having earned PhDs or MDs. RAND's areas of expertise include health, education, international relations, international development, civil and criminal justice, national security, population studies, and science and technology.

The largest single program within RAND, and the largest private health care research organization in the United States, is RAND Health. RAND Health has helped shape private- and public-sector responses to emerging health care issues for more than three decades. Our research has changed how health care is financed and delivered, in the United States and internationally, by providing evidence on:

- the effects of health insurance design and payment policies on health costs and health status
- the measurement of health care quality for physical and mental illness
- the gaps between the medical care people *should* receive and the care they *do* receive
- the cost-effectiveness of interventions to improve health care quality

Every RAND publication, database, and major briefing is carefully reviewed before its release, to ensure that the research is well-designed for the problem, based on sound information, relevant to the client's interests and needs, balanced and independent, and that the research adds value to the research area.

Additional information on RAND is available at http://www.rand.org/, and on RAND Health at http://www.rand.org/health_area/.

About RAND's Palestine Project

RAND's Center for Domestic and International Health Security (part of RAND Health) and its Center for Middle East Public Policy are undertaking an unprecedented multidisciplinary analysis of the parameters central to the success of an independent Palestinian state, over the state's first 8–10 years. The analysis includes consideration of economic, demographic, governance, education, health, public safety, security, and natural resource issues. Where appropriate, the analysis includes consideration of policy alternatives that reflect choices that might face the key participants in the process of creating such a state.

This study adopts a long-term perspective, recognizing that many short-term problems will also have to be solved in the process. It assumes that a successful Palestinian state should ultimately bring stability for Palestinians, Israelis and the region. It also assumes that substantial resources will be required from various sources in order to establish and support the institutions and infrastructure necessary for a successful independent Palestine, and it seeks to estimate the necessary resources associated with key policy alternatives. *By identifying the needs for a viable state and quantifying the costs of such a development, the parties will have a realistic appraisal of what is possible and what it will cost.*

RAND's research on Palestine is being led by a multidisciplinary team of investigators, including: Drs. Kenneth Shine and Jerrold Green (co-Project Directors),

Michael Schoenbaum (leader, Health working group), Glenn Robinson (leader, Governance working group), Robert Hunter (leader, Security working group), Jack Riley (leader, Public Safety working group), Mark Bernstein (leader, Natural Resources working group), Cheryl Benard (leader, Education working group), Brian Nichiporuk (leader, Demographics working group), and David Gompert and Richard Neu (senior advisors).

RAND's Palestine project is funded by private donations.

Additional information on RAND's Center for Domestic and International Health Security is available at http://www.rand.org/health/healthsecurity/, and on the Center for Middle East Public Policy at http://www.rand.org/nsrd/cmepp/about.html.

About RAND's Analysis of the Palestinian Health System

RAND's analysis of the Palestinian health system is being led by Drs. Michael Schoenbaum (economist, RAND), Adel Afifi (neuroscientist, University of Iowa), and Richard Deckelbaum (pediatrician and nutritionist, Columbia University); and advised by Dr. Nicole Lurie (senior natural scientist at RAND and former US Principal Deputy Assistant Secretary of Health).

The overall goals of our analysis of the Palestinian health system are: 1) to understand the strengths and gaps of the current system, with respect to organization, human and physical infrastructure, and financing; 2) to identify major priorities for future development and investment, over approximately the next ten years; and 3) to estimate the financial cost of reaching various development goals.

We recognize that there is a well-established Palestinian national health planning process. This process has led to several National Health Plans that contain detailed targets for improving health status and for developing health manpower and physical infrastructure. Evaluating each of those specific targets is outside the scope of RAND's project. At the same time, one emphasis in all the information we have gathered so far is that there is room to strengthen key Palestinian institutions, particularly relating to planning and coordination—and that such strengthening could considerably improve the health system's performance.

Our project therefore focuses on key institutions and programs that are necessary for the Palestinian health system to operate successfully, and options for strengthening these institutions. These include:

- **National health planning authority**, with responsibility for policies including division of responsibility across public, private, NGO and UNRWA sectors; authorization (certificate of need) for new buildings and expensive equipment; accreditation guidelines for providers, facilities, and education programs; clinical quality improvement; and health care finance

- **Licensing and accreditation bodies**, including for health care providers, delivery facilities, laboratories, educational programs, pharmaceuticals and medical devices
- **Policies for health insurance and finance**, including effective financing mechanisms; defined benefit and payment schedules; and incentives for quality, efficiency and health promotion
- **Prescription drug policy**, including a cost-effective national essential drugs list, policies regarding generic substitution, and efficient purchasing mechanisms
- **Health information systems**, for tracking elements including health and nutritional status, outpatient care, hospital discharges, health care quality, health system staffing, and billing and payments
- **Health manpower strategy**, including strategies to strengthen existing training programs and to meet needs that are currently unmet
- **Research and evaluation capacity**, including health policy and evaluation and biomedical research

In addition, we will examine:

- **Fast-track public and primary health care interventions**, to address current deficiencies and ensure a stable basis for population health that supports longer-term health planning

We recognize that the current security closures and travel restrictions have implications for the Palestinian health system. As above, however, the overall focus of this project is on fostering the success of a future independent Palestinian state. For purposes of this project, we therefore do *not* focus on short-term strategies for operating the health system under the current conditions. Instead, we focus on longer-term health system development, under the assumption of unrestricted travel within the West Bank and Gaza.

Planned Trip to the Region

We are preparing for a trip to Palestine and Israel in May, during which we will meet with key Palestinian, Israeli and international stakeholders regarding the Palestinian health system. *We would like to speak with you about your work, and meet if possible.* In our meetings, we will ask people to address the following issues:

1. Which health policy issues require most urgent attention? What five policy changes *can* and *should* be implemented *immediately*?

2. Based on your knowledge of the institutions described above, how well do those institutions currently function in the Palestinian health system? Which institutions particularly need to be strengthened? How could they be strengthened?
3. Have we left out any key institutions that need to be strengthened in the Palestinian health system? Which?
4. What are the major barriers that affect successful development of the Palestinian health system?

Finally, we will want to collect information on the potential costs of implementing various policy options. We will also have other questions related to your area of expertise.

We understand that other organizations are studying the Palestinian health system and providing technical assistance, including the European Union's health sector review on behalf of the Palestinian Ministry of Health. Although our mission is to conduct independent analyses, we will coordinate with these other projects as much as possible.

We will contact your office about meeting with us in May. If you have questions about this project or would like additional information, please feel free to contact any of us directly using the contact information listed above; or through our representative in Jerusalem, Ms. Timea Spitka, at <telephone number>. Thank you.

Respectfully yours,

Michael Schoenbaum, PhD	Richard Deckelbaum, MD	Adel Afifi, MD, MS
Leader, Health Working Group	Consultant	Consultant

Integration with Prior and Concurrent Health Sector Analyses

As we began this project, we learned that the European Union (EU) was sponsoring a comprehensive health sector review on behalf of the Palestinian MOH. This review is being led by the EU, with participation by the World Bank, the WHO, the British Department for International Development, the Italian Cooperation, and possibly others.

Based on draft documents about the health sector review that were provided to RAND in April 2003 and on conversations with participating organizations, we understood the general objectives of the EU health sector review to be similar to those of RAND's project—i.e., to understand the current Palestinian health system and propose options for developing the sector over the coming decade. However, the EU and RAND efforts differ on several dimensions.

The EU review is being conducted on behalf of the Ministry of Health by representatives of organizations that have also been major donors, lenders, and/or providers of technical assistance to the Palestinian health system. At present, the EU project is limited to the health sector.

RAND's review is being conducted independently, and RAND has had no involvement, advisory or otherwise, in the Palestinian health system. In addition, RAND's analysis of the health system is part of a larger, multisector study of policy options for a future Palestinian state.

Overall, however, we view the respective projects as strongly complementary. Following conversations and correspondence with the EU and other members of the review team, we agreed to pursue ongoing communication with the EU team regarding our work plan, analyses, and findings. We interviewed representatives from several of the participating organizations during our visit to Palestine and Israel in May, as listed in Appendix B. The projects have otherwise been conducted independently. Analyses for this book were scheduled to be completed before the EU health sector review.

More generally, there have been a number of previous analyses of the Palestinian health system conducted by researchers, NGOs, international donors, and of course the Palestinian Council of Health and the MOH. We recognize that most or all of the issues we address here have been addressed in previous plans and analyses. We have tried to apply an independent perspective and to build on and extend previous work to maximize the relevance of this analysis.

Bibliography

Abdeen, Z., et al., *Nutritional Assessment of the West Bank and Gaza Strip,* mimeo, Jerusalem, September 2002.

Abdeen, Z., G. Greenough, R. Qasrawi, and B. Dandies, *Nutrition & Quantitative Food Assessment, Palestinian Territories, 2003,* Jerusalem, 2004. Online at http://www.healthinforum.net/files/nutrition/Nutrion_Quant_Food_Ass03.pdf (as of October 2004).

Abdul-Rahim, H., N. Abdu-Rmeileh, et al., "Obesity and Selected Co-Morbidities in an Urban Palestinian Population," *International Journal of Obesity,* Vol. 25, 2001, pp. 1736–1740.

Abdul-Rahim, H., G. Holmboe-Ottesen, et al., "Obesity in a Rural and an Urban Palestinian West Bank Population," *International Journal of Obesity,* Vol. 27, 2003, pp. 140–146.

Abdul-Rahim, H., A. Husseini, E. Bjertness, et al., "The Metabolic Syndrome in the West Bank Population—An Urban Rural Comparison," *Diabetes Care,* Vol. 24, No. 2, February 2001, pp. 275–279.

Abdul-Rahim, H., A. Husseini, R. Giacaman, et al., "Diabetes Mellitus in an Urban Palestinian Population: Prevalence and Associated Factors," *Eastern Mediterranean Health Journal,* Vol. 7, No. 1, 2, 2001.

Afana, A. H., et al., " The Ability of General Practitioners to Detect Mental Disorders Among Primary Care Patients in a Stressful Environment: Gaza Strip," *Journal of Public Health Medicine,* Vol. 24, No. 4, December 2002, pp. 326–331.

Al-Khatib, A., and S. Salah, "Bacteriological and Chemical Quality of Swimming Pool Water in Developing Countries: A Case Study in the West Bank of Palestine," *International Journal of Environmental Health Research,* Vol. 13, 2003, pp. 17–22.

Al-Khatib, A., et al., "Water-Health Relationships in Developing Countries: A Case Study in Tulkarem District in Palestine," *International Journal of Environmental Health and Research,* Vol. 13, June 2003, pp. 199–206.

Aoyama, A., *Toward a Virtuous Circle: A Nutrition Review of the Middle East and North Africa,* Washington, D.C.: World Bank, August 1999.

Aqel N. M., et al., "Gaza's Health Services," *The Lancet,* Vol. 2, No. 8567, November 1987, pp. 1090–1091.

Arab Medical Welfare Association, *Medical Bulletin Continuing Medical Education,* Vol. 1, No. 2, Ramallah, 1999.

Arafat, C., and N. Boothby, *A Psychosocial Assessment of Palestinian Children,* Tel Aviv, Israel: USAID, 2004. Online at http://www.usaid.gov/wbg/reports/Final_CPSP_Assessment_ English.pdf (as of October 2004).

Barghouthi, M., L. Fragiacomo, and M. Qutteina, *Health Research in Palestine: An Annotated Bibliography,* 4th ed., Ramallah: Health Development Information and Policy Institute, 1999.

Barghouthi, M., A. Shubita, and L. Fragiacomo, *The Palestinian Health System: An Updated Overview,* Ramallah: Health Development Information and Policy Institute, March 2000.

Barnea, T., and R. Husseini, eds., *Separate and Cooperate, Cooperate and Separate: The Disengagement of the Palestine Health Care System from Israel and Its Emergence as an Independent System,* Westport, Conn.: Praeger, 2002.

Beckerleg, S., et al., "Purchasing a Quick Fix from Private Pharmacies in the Gaza Strip," *Social Science and Medicine,* Vol. 49, No. 1, December 1999, pp. 1489–1500.

Belgian-Israeli-Palestinian Cooperation Project in Applied Scientific Research, Training and Education, *Policies and Strategies of Future Israeli-Palestinian Academic Cooperation Draft Report on Public Health,* mimeo, November 1999.

Centers for Disease Control and Prevention (CDC), *2001 Health Data,* 2003 reprint. Online at www.cdc.gov/nchs/data/hus/tables/2003/03hus106.pdf (as of June 2004).

Cockcroft, A., *West Bank and Gaza Service Delivery Survey: Health and Basic Education Services,* Washington, D.C.: World Bank, December 1998.

de Jong, J. T., et al., "Lifetime Events and Posttraumatic Stress Disorder in 4 Postconflict Settings," *Journal of the American Medical Association,* Vol. 286, No. 5, August 1, 2001, pp. 555–562. Comment in *Journal of the American Medical Association,* Vol. 286, No. 5, August 1, 2001, pp. 584–588.

Donati, S., R. Hamam, and E. Medda, "Family Planning KAP Survey in Gaza," *Social Science and Medicine,* Vol. 50, No. 6, March 2000, pp. 841–849.

Economic Cooperation Foundation and Palestinian Council of Health, *Building Bridges Through Health, Israeli-Palestinian Cooperation in Health, Medicine and Social Welfare, 2000 Report,* February 2001.

———, *Building Bridges Through Health, Israeli-Palestinian Cooperation in Health, Medicine and Social Welfare, 1999 Report,* February 2000.

European Commission and Eurostat, *Euro-Mediterranean Statistics,* Luxembourg: European Committees, 2001.

Gaumer, G., et al., *Rationalization Plan for Hospital Beds in Egypt,* Partnerships for Health Reform Technical Report No. 29, Bethesda, Md.: Abt Associates, 1998. Online at http://www. phrplus.org/Pubs/te29fin.pdf (as of August 2003).

Giacaman, R., H. Abdul-Rahim, and L. Wick, "Health Sector Reform in the Occupied Palestinian Territories (OPT): Targeting the Forest or the Trees?" *Health Policy and Planning,* Vol. 18, No. 1, 2003, pp. 59–67.

Giacaman, R., and S. Halileh, "Maintaining Public Health Education in the West Bank," *The Lancet,* Vol. 361, No. 9364, April 2003, pp. 1220–1221.

Halileh, S., "Israeli-Palestinian Conflict. Need for Medical Services for Palestinians Injured in West Bank Is Urgent," *British Medical Journal,* Vol. 324, No. 7333, February 9, 2002, p. 361.

Halileh, S., et al., "The Impact of the Intifada on the Health of a Nation," *Medicine Conflict and Survival,* Vol. 18, No. 3, July–September 2002, pp. 239–247.

The Hashemite Kingdom of Jordan, *Human Resources,* "A Healthy Population," Jordan, 2004. Online at http://www.kinghussein.gov.jo/resources4.html (as of January 28, 2004).

Health, Development, Information, and Policy Institute (HDIP), *Coordinating Primary Health Care,* Policy Dialogues Series, No. 3, Ramallah, June 1997.

———, *The Future of Hospital Services in Palestine—A Coordination Workshop on Hospital Care,* Ramallah, September 1999.

———, *Health Care Under Siege II: The Health Situation of Palestinians During the First Two Months of the Intifada,* Ramallah, December 2000.

———, *Health Insurance and Health Service Utilization in the West Bank and Gaza Strip,* Ramallah, February 1998.

———, *Sharing Responsibility,* Policy Dialogues Series, No. 2, Ramallah, December 1996.

———, *Towards Better and Cost-Effective Hospital Care,* Policy Dialogues Series, No. 4, Ramallah, July 1998.

"Health Without Borders in the Middle East," session proceeding presented at the Annual Conference: Health and Politics in the 21st Century of the Israel National Institute for Health Policy and Health Research, Jerusalem, 2001.

Husseini, A., H. Abdul-Rahim, et al., "Prevalence of Diabetes Mellitus and Impaired Glucose Tolerance in a Rural Palestinian Population," *East Mediterranean Health Journal,* Vol. 6, No. 5–6, September–November 2000a, pp. 1039–1045.

———, "Selected Factors Associated with Diabetes Mellitus in a Rural Palestinian Community," *Medical Science Monitor,* Vol. 9, No. 5, 2003, pp. CR181–CR185.

———, "Type 2 Diabetes Mellitus, Impaired Glucose Tolerance and Associated Factors in a Rural Palestinian Village," *Diabetic Medicine,* Vol. 17, 2000b, pp. 746–748.

———, "The Utility of a Single Glucometer Measurement of Fasting Capillary Blood Glucose in the Prevalence Determination of Diabetes Mellitus in an Urban Adult Palestinian Population," *Scand J Lab Invest,* Vol. 60, 2000c, pp. 457–462.

"In Shift, U.S. to Aid the Palestinian Authority," *The New York Times,* Late Edition—Final, July 8, 2003, Sec. A, p. 6.

International Crisis Group, *Islamic Social Welfare Activism in the Occupied Palestinian Territories: A Legitimate Target?* International Crisis Group Middle East Report No. 13, Amman/Brussels, 2003.

Khamis, V., *Political Violence and the Palestine Family: Implications for Mental Health and Well-Being*, mimeo, 2000.

Lennock, M., *Health in Palestine: Potential and Challenges*, mimeo, March 1997.

Lewando-Hundt, G., Y. Abed, M. Skeik, S. Beckerleg, and A. El Alem, "Addressing Birth in Gaza: Using Qualitative Methods to Improve Vital Registration," *Social Science and Medicine*, Vol. 48, No. 6, March 1999, pp. 833–843.

Lilienfield, L., J. Rose, and M. Corn, "UNRWA and the Health of Palestinian Refugees. United Nations Relief and Works Agency," *New England Journal of Medicine*, Vol. 315, No. 9, August 28, 1986, pp. 595–600.

Madi, H., "Infant and Child Mortality Rates Among Palestinian Refugee Populations," *The Lancet*, Vol. 356, No. 9226, July 22, 2000, p. 312.

Massoud, R. F., "A Study of the Financial Statement of Health for the West Bank and Gaza," Harvard School of Public Health, Harvard University, mimeo, 1993.

Medistat, *Medistat—Country Profiles, Egypt*, West Sussex, U.K.: Medistat, Espicom Business Intelligence, April 2003. Online at http://www.espicom.com/web.nsf/structure/TocsMedistat01/$File/egypt.PDF (as of February 2004).

Organisation for Economic Co-operation and Development (OECD), *OECD Health Data 2004*, 1st edition, Paris: Organisation for Economic Co-operation and Development, 2004.

———, *OECD Health Data 1997*, Paris: Organisation for Economic Co-operation and Development, 1997.

———, *Requirements and Guidelines for the Accreditation of Nursing Education Programs in Palestine*, April 1996.

Palestine Red Crescent Society, *Operating Under Siege*, Ramallah, January 2001–December 2002.

Palestinian Authority, *Palestinian Development Plan, 1999–2003*, January 1999.

Palestinian Authority, Palestinian Council of Health, and PA MOH, *The Strategic Plan for Quality of Health Care in Palestine*, mimeo, December 1994.

Palestinian Authority Ministry of Health (PA MOH), *Health Indicators, Palestine 2002*, July 2003a. Online at http://www.healthinforum.net/files/moh_reports/Health Indicators 2002.pdf (as of July 2003).

———, *Health Status in Palestine, Annual Report 2001*, July 2002a.

———, *National Strategic Health Plan, 1999–2003*, 1999.

———, *Nutrition Strategies in Palestine*, July 2003b.

———, *Palestine National Cancer Registry—Cancer Incidence in Palestine 1998–1999*, December 2001.

———, *Palestinian Drug Formulary*, 1st ed., 2002b.

———, *The Status of Health in Palestine*, 1998.

———, *The Status of Health in Palestine: Annual Report*, June 1997.

Palestinian Authority Ministry of Health and Al-Quds University, *Report on Iodine Deficiency Survey in West Bank and Gaza Strip*, April 1997.

Palestinian Authority and the United Nations Children's Fund, *The Situation Analysis of Palestinian Children, Young People & Women in the West Bank and Gaza Strip*, August 2000.

Palestinian Central Bureau of Statistics, *Health Survey 2000—Executive Summary*, November 2000a.

Palestinian Council of Health, *The Nursing Human Resource in Palestine*, January 1997.

Palestinian Council of Health, et al., *Palestinian-Israeli Cooperation in Developing Occupational Health and Safety Services in Palestine*, February 2000.

Palestinian Council of Health, Planning and Research Centre, *The National Health Plan for the Palestinian People: Objectives and Strategies*, Jerusalem, April 1994.

———, *Workshop Proceedings: Regional Workshop on Substance Abuse*, October 1999.

———, *Health Survey 2000, Main Findings*, November 2000b.

———, *Nutrition Survey 2002—Press Conference on the Survey Results*, 2002.

Partnerships for Health Reform, *Jordan Embarks on Health System Reform to Preserve Health Gains and Expand Coverage*, Jordan: Partnerships for Health Reform, September 1997. Online at http://www.phrplus.org/Pubs/pib10.pdf (as of February 2004).

Primary Health Care Preventive Medicine Department, *Palestine Annual Communicable Disease Report*, Ramallah, 1999.

Ramlawi, A., *Preventive Medicine Team. Brucellosis Prevention and Control Program: (KAP) Knowledge—Attitude and Practice in Palestine*, Palestinian Authority Ministry of Health, 2000a.

———, *Preventive Medicine Team. Viral Hepatitis Survey 2000*, Palestinian Authority Ministry of Health, 2000b.

Reinhardt, U. E., P. S. Hussey, and G. F. Anderson, "Cross-National Comparisons of Health Systems Using OECD Data 1999, *Health Affairs* (Millwood), Vol. 21, No. 3, May–June 2002, pp. 169–181.

Schnitzer, J., and S. Roy, "Health Services in Gaza Under the Autonomy Plan," *The Lancet*, Vol. 343, No. 8913, June 1994, pp. 1614–1617. Comments in *The Lancet*, Vol. 344, No. 8920, August 1994, p. 478; *The Lancet*, Vol. 343, No. 8913, June 1994, pp. 1581–1582.

Schoenbaum, M., T. Tulchinsky, and Y. Abed, "Gender Differences in Nutritional Status and Feeding Patterns Among Infants in the Gaza Strip," *American Journal of Public Health*, Vol. 85, No. 7, July 1995, pp. 965–969.

Shani, M., and T. Tulchinsky, "Health in Gaza," *British Medical Journal*, Vol. 307, No. 6902, August 21, 1993, p. 509. Comment in *British Medical Journal*, Vol. 308, No. 6921, January 8, 1994, p. 137.

Stene L., R. Giacaman, H. Abdul-Rahim, A. Husseini, K. Norum, and G. Holmboe-Ottesen, "Food Consumption Pattern in a Palestinian West Bank Population," *European Journal of Clinical Nutrition*, Vol. 53, 1999, pp. 953–958.

————, "Obesity and Associated Factors in a Palestinian West Bank Village Population," *European Journal of Clinical Nutrition,* Vol. 55, 2001, pp. 805–811.

Thabet, A. A., Y. Abed, and P. Vostanis, "Emotional Problems in Palestinian Children Living in a War Zone: A Cross-Sectional Study, *The Lancet,* Vol. 359, No. 9320, May 25, 2002, pp. 1801–1804. Comments in *The Lancet,* Vol. 359, No. 9320, May 25, 2002, pp. 1793–1794; *The Lancet,* Vol. 360, No. 9339, October 5, 2002, p. 1098; *The Lancet,* Vol. 361, No. 9353, January 18, 2003, p. 260.

Tulchinsky, T. H., "Medical Services in Gaza," *The Lancet,* Vol. 1, No. 8530, February 1987, p. 450.

Tulchinsky, T. H., Y. Abed, G. Ginsberg, S. Shaheen, J. Friedman, M. Schoenbaum, and P. Slater, "Measles in Israel, the West Bank and Gaza: Continuing Incidence and the Case for a New Eradication Strategy," *Reviews of Infectious Diseases,* Vol. 12, 1990, pp. 951–958.

Tulchinsky, T. H., Y. Abed, S. Shaheen, N. Toubassi, Y. Sever, M. Schoenbaum, and R. Handsher, "A Ten Year Experience in Control of Poliomyelitis Through a Combination of Live and Killed Vaccines in Two Developing Areas," *American Journal of Public Health,* Vol. 79, No. 12, December 1989, pp. 1648–1652.

Tulchinsky, T. H., A. M. Al Zeer, J. Abu Mounshar, T. Subeih, M. Schoenbaum, et al., "A Successful, Preventive-Oriented Village Health Worker Program in Hebron, the West Bank, 1985–1996," *Journal of Public Health Management and Practice,* Vol. 3, No. 4, 1997, pp. 57–67.

Tulchinsky, T. H., S. El Ebweini, G. M. Ginsberg, Y. Abed, D. Montano-Cuellar, M. Schoenbaum, et al., "Growth and Nutrition Patterns of Infants in Association with a Nutrition Education/Supplementation Program in Gaza, 1987–1992," *Bulletin of the World Health Organization,* Vol. 72, 1994, pp. 869–875.

Tulchinsky, T. H., and J. Shemer, "Health Services in Gaza Under the Autonomy Plan," *The Lancet,* Vol. 344, No. 8920, August 1994, p. 478. Comment in *The Lancet,* Vol. 343, No. 8913, June 1994, pp. 1614–1617.

United Nations Children's Fund, *The State of the World's Children,* New York, 2000. Online at http://www.unicef.org/sowc00/ (as of February 2004).

United Nations Office for the Coordination of Humanitarian Affairs, "Humanitarian Monitoring Report: Commitments Made by the Government of Israel to Ms. Catherine Bertini, Personal Humanitarian Envoy to the Middle East for the Secretary General," Jerusalem, June 2003. Online at http://www.healthinforum.net/files/misc/Humanitarian%20Monitoring%20Report-June03.pdf (as of February 2004).

United Nations Relief and Works Agency for Palestine Refugees in the Near East, *Annual Report of the Department of Health,* Amman, Jordan, 2001.

The United States Agency for International Development (USAID) West Bank and Gaza, *Health and Humanitarian Assistance Portfolio Overview,* Washington, D.C.: USAID, May 22, 2003.

Welfare Association, Palestinian Authority, and Ministry of Higher Education, *National Plan for Human Resource Development and Education in Health, Overview Volume,* Jerusalem: Welfare Association, 2001a.

————, *National Plan for Human Resource Development and Education in Health, Report #1: Planning, Accreditation and Licensure of Health Professionals in Palestine: Suggested Models,* Jerusalem: Welfare Association, 2001b.

————, *National Plan for Human Resource Development and Education in Health, Report #2: Appraisal of Palestinian Educational Programs in Health,* Jerusalem: Welfare Association, 2001c.

————, *National Plan for Human Resource Development and Education in Health, Report #3: Appraisal of CE [Continuing Education] Infrastructure in Major Health Service Provider Organizations in Palestine,* Jerusalem: Welfare Association, 2001d.

————, *National Plan for Human Resource Development and Education in Health, Report #4: Appraisal of CE [Continuing Education] Needs of Graduates of Educational Programs and Practicing Professionals in Health,* Jerusalem: Welfare Association, 2001e.

————, *National Plan for Human Resource Development and Education in Health, Report #5: Professionals, Sub Plans,* Jerusalem: Welfare Association, 2001f.

World Bank, *Competitiveness Indicators,* 2003a. Online at http://wbln0018.worldbank.org/psd/compete.nsf/ (as of August 2003).

————, *Project Appraisal on a Proposed Credit in the Amount of US$7.9 Million to West Bank and Gaza for a Health System Development Project,* Washington, D.C., November 8, 1999.

————, *West Bank and Gaza: Medium-Term Development Strategy for the Health Sector,* Washington, D.C., August 1998.

————, *World Development Indicators 2003,* CD-ROM, Washington, D.C., 2003b.

World Food Program (WFP), *Emergency Food Security Needs Assessment: 2004 Update Assessment,* Jerusalem, Israel: World Food Program 2004. Online at http://documents.wfp.org/stellent/groups/public/documents/ena/wfp036508.pdf (as of October 2004).

World Health Organization (WHO), *Country Statistics, United States,* Geneva, Switzerland: World Health Organization Headquarters, 2001.

————, *Essential Drugs and Medicine Policy,* "WHO Model List of Essential Drugs," 11th ed., Geneva, Switzerland: World Health Organization Headquarters, 1999. Online at http://www.who.int/medicines/organization/par/edl/infedl11alpha.html (as of February 2004).

————, *Essential Drugs and Medicine Policy,* "The WHO Model List of Essential Medicines," 12th ed., Geneva, Switzerland: World Health Organization Headquarters, 2002. Online at http://www.who.int/medicines/organization/par/edl/eml12.shtml (as of February 2004).

————, *European Health-for-All Database,* Copenhagen, Denmark: World Health Organization, Regional Office for Europe, 2004. Online at http://hfadb.who.dk/hfa/(as of February 2004).

————, *Severe Mobility Restrictions in West Bank and Gaza Force Palestinian Population to Change Health Services,* press release, Jerusalem: WHO Office for the West Bank and Gaza, August 2003a. Online at http://www.healthinforum.net/modules.php?name = News&file = article&sid = 118 (as of February 2004).

————, *Survey on Access to Health Services in the Occupied Palestinian Territories—Preliminary Results and Comments,* Jerusalem: WHO Office for the West Bank and Gaza, August 2003b.